SACRA
WITHDRA
SA
CIRCU

D0207447

The Sleeved Life

A Patient-to-Patient Guide on Vertical Sleeve
Gastrectomy Weight Loss Surgery

Pennie Nicola

Copyright © 2012 Pennie Nicola

All rights reserved.

ISBN-10: 1475179693
ISBN-13: 978-1475179699

CONTENTS

Vertical Sleeve Gastrectomy

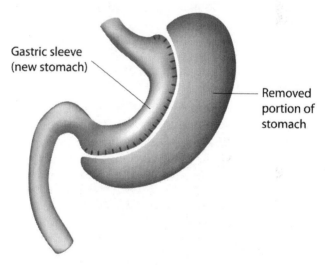

Gastric sleeve
(new stomach)

Removed
portion of
stomach

FORWARD

If you are reading this book, you have likely either recently had, or are considering, vertical sleeve gastrectomy weight loss surgery. This book is intended to be a helpful guide for you in your journey, both in making this life-changing decision and in living the "sleeved life." **I am not a medical expert or a doctor.** I am a patient battling obesity with the help of a powerful tool called the vertical sleeve.

Vertical sleeve gastrectomy is still a relatively new bariatric procedure. When I started my journey, I could find no other patients who had this surgery. I knew of many with the gastric bypass or the adjustable band, but no sleeve patients. Even today, my support group meetings consist almost entirely of gastric bypass and adjustable band patients. I have found a larger network of support online, and I've been able to connect with other sleeve patients all over the world. I wanted to write this book so that patients considering the sleeve surgery or patients who have recently had the sleeve surgery could hear from a fellow "sleever." I had so many questions I wanted to ask a sleeve patient before I had my surgery, and I hope this book might help fill that void for other patients.

I hope this book is a helpful companion. Please remember the contents are coming from a fellow patient and **nothing in this book is to be taken as medical advice**. I hope you find this book of questions and answers about the sleeve surgery helpful on your own journey.

Best,

Pennie Nicola

CHAPTER 1
IS WEIGHT LOSS SURGERY RIGHT FOR ME?

Is weight loss surgery right for me? This is really the biggest question in this book of questions. It's a difficult one to answer, so I thought I'd try to shed some light on this issue with a story.

It was a crisp Midwestern fall day and about 40 obese people were sitting in a small conference room at a hospital. The room was quiet except for the occasional cough or rustling of papers. A thin woman wearing a white lab coat entered the conference room and walked to the podium at the front.

"Good afternoon," she said brightly. "I'm glad you could make it today. This could be the first day of your journey to a healthier life."

The hospital hosted these informational meetings once a month. They were free to anyone interested in learning more about weight loss surgery. The nurse gave a PowerPoint presentation that provided an overview of the different surgeries and what was expected of patients before and after surgery. At the end of the presentation, she asked if anyone had any questions.

At first, no one said a word or even moved a muscle. Perhaps we were a room full of introverts or perhaps we were all still just absorbing the massive amount of information that had been presented. Finally, a middle-aged woman with an oxygen tank resting beside her legs raised her hand.

"Can I still drink soda?" she asked.

"No," the nurse said. "You'll need to give up soda during the pre-op diet."

"Why can't I have soda?" the woman asked, sounding a bit upset.

"The carbonation isn't good for your pouch, not to mention the empty calories aren't going to help you with weight loss," the nurse answered.

"What if I let it go flat first?" the woman persisted.

"No," the nursed sighed, but continued to smile politely. "If you have weight loss surgery you will need to make a lot of lifestyle changes. Giving up soda is just one of them."

The woman shook her head and muttered something that I couldn't hear. She was clearly very unhappy about this answer.

As the meeting continued, more people asked questions about what they could and couldn't eat after surgery. People asked how much weight they could expect to lose. A few people asked about insurance requirements, support groups, and if they'd have to count calories.

"If no one else has any more questions," the nurse said, turning off the projector that had displayed the PowerPoint presentation on the wall behind her, "the next step is to schedule an appointment for a consultation."

There was another nurse waiting outside the conference room with a laptop on a folding table. She was the next step, scheduling the appointment to meet with the surgeon and his team of bariatric experts to determine if weight loss surgery is the best course of treatment.

I had researched weight loss surgery for three years before coming to this meeting. I had talked to a couple of other surgeons. I had read every scientific paper I could find. I understood what would be expected of me before and after surgery well before I saw the PowerPoint presentation. I felt I was ready. About half of the people in the conference room came out and also joined me in line to take the next step. They too had decided they were ready.

The people who did not get in line filed out of the conference room and walked past us. For more reasons that I could possibly list here, they decided that surgery wasn't right for them or that they just weren't ready yet.

One of the last to leave the conference room was the woman with the oxygen tank, the woman who didn't want to give up soda. Her mobility was limited; she shuffled slowly out the door, pulling her small tank of oxygen behind her. I saw she had a motorized wheelchair waiting for her, parked a few feet away from the conference room door. It was too wide to fit through the doorway, so she had to leave it outside the conference room. She looked up at the line of 20 or so people waiting to make an appointment with the nurse and shook her head.

"I can't give up soda," she said to none of us in particular. "I just can't do it."

Some people smiled and nodded at her sympathetically, but one man decided to speak up.

"Of course you can," he said. "It would be worth it. Once you'd start losing weight, you'd never look back."

"I drink 8 sodas a day and I have since I was a kid," the woman said as she eased herself onto her scooter. She sighed and looked up at the man. Her voiced began to sound defensive. "I've tried to give it up before, and I can't. I wish I had known that you couldn't have soda after weight loss surgery or I wouldn't have wasted my time here."

The man didn't say anything. One of the ladies in line behind him said "goodbye" to the woman with the oxygen tank as she exited down the hallway towards the elevators. The woman didn't respond.

Weight loss surgery isn't for everyone. Even for those who could benefit from weight loss surgery, it may not be their best solution. Weight loss surgery requires a great deal of rule compliance, and if someone isn't mentally or emotionally ready for the drastic changes that weight loss surgery requires, then it isn't the best solution for him or her.

I still sometimes think about the woman with the oxygen tank. I don't know if soda was really the issue or if she was looking for a reason to not have weight loss surgery. The reasons we choose to have or not have surgery are very complicated and very personal. If she knew that she couldn't give up soda, she was very wise to not have surgery. She would be at risk of hurting herself if she couldn't stick to the rules laid out for her in the program. I hope she has found something that works for her. Her mobility and health would be likely to continue to deteriorate if she didn't act right away.

Now, fast forward, and I've had the vertical sleeve gastrectomy (or "sleeve") surgery. I attend support group meetings twice a month filled with people who have had, or are about to have, weight loss surgery. Most of the people in my support group have the gastric bypass, several with adjustable gastric banding and just a couple of others, like me, with the sleeve. How did we all decide that surgery was right for us when the vast majority of morbidly obese people choose to not have surgery?

Our reasons vary, of course. One thing we all seem to have in common is that we've all tried almost every diet under the sun. We've done shakes; we've done cabbage soup; we've done low fat, low carb, low calories; we've done meal delivery services; we've tried diet pills; we've tried intensive exercise; we've tried almost every infomercial for the latest-greatest weight loss product out there. Despite all of these efforts, we have all failed....or, perhaps, these efforts have failed *us*.

Some of us have been obese since childhood; some gained weight later in life. Most of us have lost weight, even significant amounts of weight, but none of us has kept it off successfully. In fact, most of us gain back all of the weight we lose and then a little extra too.

How did you know that weight loss surgery was the best choice?

For me, personally, I knew weight loss surgery was the right solution before I was even ready for it. My reasoning was rather academic. I knew that once someone reaches the "morbidly obese" category—which is a BMI of 40 or more—diet and exercise is more likely to fail to than to work. In fact, the success rate of long-term weight loss maintenance with lifestyle changes ranges from 2–20% (Wing & Phelan, 2005. Long-term weight loss maintenance. *American Journal of Clinical Nutrition* **82**[1], 207S–273S). The lowest success rate is associated with the higher starting weights. Morbidly obese people have a 95-98% failure rate when it comes to diet and exercise. Some weight can be lost, but it doesn't usually stay off.

Weight loss surgery isn't perfect. It has risks, serious risks, that must be considered carefully... but the success rate is much better. In fact, bariatric surgery is the single most effective treatment for morbid obesity available today. My surgeon shared with me that his practice has a 95% success rate with sleeve patients. While national data isn't quite as impressive, contributors to the 3rd International Summit for Sleeve Gastrectomy recently reported that five years after sleeve surgery, patients had maintained a weight loss of 60% of their excess weight. To me, weight loss surgery seemed like the obvious solution after 20 years of yo-yo dieting and only morbid obesity and a host of related health problems to show for it. Weight loss surgery gave me better odds.

How is "success" defined when it comes to statistics?

This is a very important question to ask anytime you are given a success rate— whether from your surgeon or from a diet program. In the world of bariatric surgery, it's generally agreed that success is defined as keeping off at least 50% of your excess weight. Of course, most patients hope to lose more than 50% of their excess weight—and the majority do so!

How did you decide you were "ready" for weight loss surgery?

For me, learning about the impressive statistics and hearing success stories wasn't enough. I still wasn't ready. I was ready for the lifestyle change. I wasn't worried about giving up soda or any other forbidden fruit. I was, after all, an expert dieter. Most of my life had been a cycle of dietary deprivation followed by periods of excess. My problem was that I wasn't too sold on the two most popular weight loss surgeries offered at the time: the gastric bypass and the adjustable-band. It wasn't until the sleeve became an option that I was finally *ready* for weight loss surgery. Once I learned that a respected local surgeon was performing sleeve surgeries, I knew my time had come.

Am I a candidate for weight loss surgery?

I think when determining if weight loss surgery is right for you, you first have to start with the question "Do I qualify?" Not everyone qualifies for weight loss surgery. Most surgeons and insurance companies require that patients have a starting BMI of 40 or greater. You may also qualify if you have a BMI of 35 or greater as long as you have one or two co-morbidites. A co-morbidity is a medical condition that is caused or exacerbated by your obesity—such as hypertension or sleep apnea. You can easily calculate your BMI using an online calculator such as the one at www.nhlbisupport.com/bmi. Check with your insurance company to get details on the requirements.

Is weight loss surgery worth the risk?

Qualifying for weight loss surgery is just the first hurdle. The bigger hurdle is determining if you are willing to accept the risk of surgery and are willing to have a complete lifestyle change. Being successful means being compliant with the "rules" of post-op life. You have to be diligent with your eating, your exercise, and your medical follow-up with your surgeon for the rest of your life. If you aren't diligent, your risk for complications skyrockets. I'll talk more about risks of weight loss surgery in the next chapter.

Will weight loss surgery help with my emotional eating problems?

Perhaps one of the most important things to remember about weight loss surgery is that *it is abdominal surgery, not brain surgery*. In other words, weight loss surgery won't fix your urge to comfort or reward yourself with food; it won't stop you from eating to the point of discomfort; it won't stop you from grazing on unhealthy foods all day long. Weight loss surgery does not correct any mental or emotional reasons for overeating.

Horror stories abound about people who had weight loss surgery without addressing a pre-existing binge or compulsive eating disorder first. If you think you might be a compulsive overeater, or if you have any significant issue with food, it is in your best interest to address these issues *before* surgery. Many insurance companies require a 6-month doctor supervised diet before surgery. Take this time to enlist the help of a therapist specializing in eating disorders. Be honest with your surgeon about your food issues and do not proceed with your surgery until you are certain they are under control.

Most bariatric surgeons, especially those working at a site designated as a "Center of Excellence" by the American Society for Metabolic and Bariatric Surgery, work with psychologists not just to screen potential candidates for surgery, but also to help them work through a variety of pre- and post-operative issues. These psychologists may be on staff with the weight loss surgery center, or they might work independently but accept referrals from the surgeon.

I've decided I want to proceed with weight loss surgery, but I still have doubts. What should I do?

Once you've made the decision to have weight loss surgery, you may go through times of doubt and worry. This is major surgery and a major lifestyle change—it wouldn't be normal if you weren't a little nervous! Take the time to research and get all of your questions answered before surgery. I hope this book will be a helpful place to start, but you should also prepare a list of questions for your surgeon, read up on the latest research in medical journals (many are available online), and attend support groups to meet other people who have had the surgery.

How will I know when I've made the right decision about sleeve surgery?

You will only know in hindsight. The decision to have, or not have, weight loss surgery must be made between you and your trusted physician. This life-altering surgery has serious risks. In addition to the general risks reviewed in this book, there are many particular risks that relate to your specific health issues and history. Once you have discussed surgery with a trusted doctor and researched the issue to your satisfaction, I think if you can answer this question honestly and comfortably, then you will know what decision is right for you: *Do you firmly believe your health is at greater risk __with__ the sleeve surgery or __without__?* Once I realized that I believed the risks of not having weight loss surgery were higher than the risks of having weight loss surgery, I knew was ready.

CHAPTER 2
WHAT ARE MY SURGERY OPTIONS?

There are four types of weight loss surgery most commonly performed today: gastric bypass (Roux-en Y), adjustable gastric band, duodenal switch, and vertical sleeve gastrectomy. There are also a handful of more rarely performed surgeries, such as gastric plication.

What is gastric bypass?

When you tell someone you are considering, or have had, weight loss surgery the person will probably assume you mean gastric bypass. The term "gastric bypass" is actually used to describe any surgery that divides the stomach into a small pouch and then rearranges the small intestines. When I use the term "gastric bypass" in this book, and in conversation, I am referring to a specific type of gastric bypass surgery called the Roux-en-Y (RNY). The RNY gastric bypass is what most people mean when they say "gastric bypass."

As of the writing of this book, the majority of weight loss surgeries performed in the United States are RNY gastric bypass procedures. The RNY is a very popular surgery with a high success rate and the data to back it up. The long-term mortality rate of RNY patients is reduced by up to 40%! (Adams, Gress, Smith *et al.*, 2007. Long-term mortality after gastric bypass surgery. New England Journal of Medicine **357**[8], 753–61; Sjöström, Narbro, Sjöström *et al.*, 2007. Effects of bariatric surgery on mortality in Swedish obese subjects. *New England Journal of Medicine* **357**[8], 741–52). Most patients lose 65-80% of their excess weight.

These wonderful statistics do come with a risk. In addition to a long list of possible non-life threatening complications, approximately 0.5% of RNY patients die within a year of surgery from complications related to surgery (Complications and costs for obesity surgery declining. Agency for Healthcare Research and Quality. April 29, 2009). This statistic is relatively similar for all forms of weight loss surgery, not just gastric bypass.

With statistics like this, however, you have to keep something in mind. First, people that need to get weight loss surgery aren't usually in great health. They are high-risk patients. Second, it's hard to know how many patients would have died within a year from obesity-related complications had they NOT had weight loss surgery. I don't say this to minimize the very real life-threatening risks of bariatric surgery but rather to help keep these statistics in perspective.

It should be noted that the 0.5% mortality rate is a national average; it isn't an actual average for any given surgeon. Every surgeon has his/her own statistics. Some surgeons may have a 1% mortality rate and some may have a 0% mortality rate. This statistic alone doesn't tell the whole story as the 1% surgeon may be willing to take on super morbidly obese patients or patients who are otherwise higher risk.

How is the body altered with gastric bypass surgery?

With RNY surgery, the stomach is divided into two parts. The upper part of the stomach is separated from the rest and formed into a small pouch. This pouch is then connected to the small intestines. The small pouch is the patient's new stomach, through which all of his or her food will pass. The remaining part of the stomach is left behind, and it continues to make gastric juices that enter the intestines. It is considered to be a "blind stomach", meaning it cannot be scoped to check for ulcers or other issues.

The new stomach, the "pouch," is very small. It can only hold about 1–2 tablespoons at a time. With the gastric bypass, your new little stomach doesn't have a pyloric value. That part of your natural stomach is in the "blind stomach." The pyloric valve is the valve between the stomach and the small intestines. It regulates the release of stomach contents into the intestines for further digestion. Because the pouch doesn't have a natural pyloric valve, the surgeon creates a man-made one.

The pouch is connected to the middle portion of the small intestine, called the jejunum. This, in effect, bypasses the upper portion of the small intestine, called the duodenum. Because food is passing through less intestines, fewer calories and nutrients are absorbed into the body. This is called malabsorption.

With a smaller stomach, and the malabsorption of foods, it's easy to see why gastric bypass is an effective weight loss surgery. It has recently come to light, however, that these are not the only mechanisms that promote weight loss. A recent study (conducted with rats) showed that the gastric bypass also increases calorie expenditure while at rest— something that probably doesn't happen with the restrictive only procedures such as the sleeve or banding. In this rat study, there was a 31% increase in resting calorie expenditure in gastric bypass rats but no increase at all in rats with sleeves (Stylopoulos, Hoppin, Kaplan, & Lee, 2009. Roux-en-Y gastric bypass enhances energy expenditure and extends lifespan in diet-induced obese rats. *Obesity* **17**[10], 1839–1847). As you can see, we are still learning the way these surgeries work on our bodies and the mechanisms by which they cause weight loss!

What are the risks of gastric bypass?

Every weight loss surgery has the potential for complications, some extremely serious. The following is a list of potential complications from the RNY gastric bypass, but it isn't an exhaustive list. It's important to talk to your surgeon about potential complications and the probability of these risks in your particular case.

Immediate Surgery Risks:
- Severe bleeding
- Complications of anesthesia
- Infections
- Respiratory problems
- Blood clots
- Gastrointestinal leaks
- Death (rare)

Long Term Risks:
- Bowel obstruction
- Hypoglycemia, or reactive hypoglycemia
- Dumping syndrome (diarrhea, nausea, vomiting)
(Note: Many RNY patients see this as a plus! Dumping syndrome can usually be avoided by avoiding sugary foods. So it's motivation to stay on a strict diet!)
- Gallstones
- Vomiting
- Hernia
- Malnutrition, vitamin deficiencies
- Ulcers
- Death (rare)

What is the adjustable band?

While many people call the gastric adjustable band a "lap band." LAP BAND® is actually a specific name brand for an adjustable gastric band. Another name brand is the Realize® band. The Lap-Band System obtained FDA approval in 2001, the Realize® band in 2007.

Adjustable gastric banding is a popular procedure in which an inflatable silicone band is placed around the top portion of the stomach to restrict the amount of food the patient can eat. The band creates a "pouch" at the top of the stomach. This pouch can only hold a small amount of food. This restricts the amount of food a patient can eat in one sitting, which usually results in a reduction of calories consumed, which leads to weight loss.

The band can be "filled" and "unfilled" with a saline solution to decrease and increase the circumference and, thereby, increase and decrease the restriction. It is filled and unfilled through a port in the patient's abdomen. The patient must go to the bariatric surgeon's office in order to get his or her band adjusted.

While other forms of bariatric surgery require a BMI of 40 or more (or 35 with comorbidities), in February 2011, the FDA in the United States expanded approval of adjustable gastric band for patients with a BMI of 30 and at least one co-morbidity. The adjustable band, therefore, offers a surgical weight loss tool for some people that wouldn't otherwise qualify for weight loss surgery.

Many patients view banding as the least invasive of all the bariatric surgeries because no organs are removed or rearranged. The band is simply placed around the stomach. Like most bariatric surgeries, the adjustable band is placed using laparoscopic surgery techniques.

Other advantages to adjustable banding include the following: there is no cutting or stapling of the stomach; recovery is fairly quick; the band can be adjusted; and there are none of the malabsorption issues seen with intestinal bypass operations. Many cite the fact that the adjustable band is removable as an advantage; however such a procedure can be complicated. Adhesions sometimes form and make removal or revision a more complicated surgery.

What are the risks of adjustable gastric banding?

Every weight loss surgery has the potential for complications, some extremely serious. The following is a list of potential complications from adjustable gastric banding, but this isn't an exhaustive list. It's important to talk to your surgeon about potential complications and the probability of these risks in your particular case.

Immediate Surgery Risks:
- Severe bleeding
- Complications of anesthesia
- Infections
- Respiratory problems

- Blood clots
- Death (rare)

Long Term Risks:
- Vomiting
- Food getting "stuck" in the narrow passage between the pouch and the rest of the stomach
- Ulcers
- Gallstones
- Erosion: This happens when the band slowly erodes through the stomach wall and it can cause severe problems (Maggard, Shugarman, Suttorp et al. 2007. LAP BAND diet guidelines. University of California, San Diego; UCSD Medical Center, Center for the Treatment of Obesity, San Diego, CA; American Society of Metabolic & Bariatric Surgery, 200.)
- Band slippage. The band may slip and part of the lower stomach will prolapse through the band and into the pouch. This can cause an enlarged pouch, or in severe cases, it can cause an obstruction.
- Port flipping. There can be problems with the port or the tube connecting the port and the band. The part can potentially flip, making it inaccessible to a needle for fills and unfills.
- Removal or revisions operations
- Death (rare)

What is vertical sleeve gastrectomy?

The vertical sleeve gastrectomy (or just "sleeve" as I like to call it) is a restrictive-only bariatric surgery.

Like the gastric bypass, it is generally only available to those with a BMI of 40 or greater (or 35 and greater with comorbidities).

While it is rapidly gaining popularity, there are still fewer sleeve surgeries performed than adjustable band surgery or gastric bypass. It is relatively new as a stand-alone procedure, but it used to be done as the first step in a two-part duodenal switch operation. Super morbidly obese patients would complete the first step of the duodenal switch operation (the sleeve part) but then loose sufficient weight that they did not continue with the second part of the procedure (the intestinal bypass). In recent years, more insurance companies have agreed to include the vertical sleeve gastrectomy in their bariatric surgery coverage, and more surgeons are offering it as an option.

The surgery itself is simple. Using laparoscopic surgical techniques, the surgeon removes 75-90% of the patient's stomach. The portion of the stomach that is removed is the "greater curvature" and what is left behind resembles a long skinny banana or sleeve. It is not reversible as once the stomach is removed it cannot be replaced.

One advantage that many patients discuss with the sleeve is that the pyloric valve remains intact. Unlike the gastric bypass, in which a small pouch is created with an artificial stoma to empty food from the pouch to the intestines, with the sleeve, the patient keeps the natural pyloric valve.

Another benefit of the sleeve surgery is that it greatly reduces the amount of ghrelin in the body. This is also known as the "hunger hormone" and much of it is produced by the stomach. Once most of the stomach is removed, ghrelin levels drop. What is the result, at least theoretically? You don't feel hungry.

Surgeons often use a "bougie" to help guide the size of the stomach, which range in size from 32-60 French. The small sleeve is usually approximately 15 mL in size (Karmali, 2010. Laparoscopic sleeve gastrectomy: an innovative new tool in the battle against the obesity epidemic in Canada. *Canadian Journal of Surgery* **53**(2):126-32.)

What are the risks of vertical sleeve gastrectomy?

Every weight loss surgery has the potential for complications, some extremely serious. The following is a list of potential complications from the vertical sleeve surgery, but it isn't an exhaustive list. It's important to talk to your surgeon about potential complications and the probability of these risks in your particular case.

Immediate Surgery Risks:
- Severe bleeding
- Complications of anesthesia
- Infections
- Respiratory problems
- Blood clots
- Stomach leaks

- Death (rare)

Long Term Risks:
- Gallstones
- Vomiting
- Hernia
- Ulcers
- Death (rare)

What is duodenal switch?

The duodenal switch is arguably the most powerful weight loss surgery performed today. It is also one of the least commonly performed. It combines the restriction of a sleeved-stomach with the malabsorption of intestinal re-routing. Patients with the duodenal switch malabsorb more calories than gastric bypass patients. They also appear to keep a degree of calorie malabsorption the rest of their lives (unlike gastric bypass patient who keep nutrient malabsorption but eventually begin to absorb most calories eaten again). Their sleeved stomachs are typically a bit larger than the sleeved stomachs of patients who have a vertical sleeve gastrectomy.

The duodenal switch is a powerful combination of restriction and malabsorption which successfully produces a high weight loss with very little weight regain. (Prachand Davee, & Alverdy, 2006. Duodenal switch provides superior weight loss in the super-obese [BMI > or =50 kg/m2] compared with gastric bypass. *Annals of Surgery* **244**(4), 611–9).

Furthermore, the duodenal switch boasts a 98-99% cure rate for type 2 diabetes (Hess, Hess, & Oakley, 2005. The biliopancreatic diversion with the duodenal switch: Results beyond 10 years. *Obesity Surgery* **15**(3), 408–16; Baltasar, Bou, Bengochea, Arlandis, Escriva, Mir, Martinez, & Perez, 2001. Duodenal switch: An effective therapy for morbid obesity—intermediate results. *Obesity Surgery* **11**(1), 54–8). If a patient decides he or she wants the duodenal switch, the patient will find that most bariatric surgeons do not offer this type of surgery. You will need to seek out an experienced surgeon, one who performs this complicated operation regularly.

Despite the impressive weight loss and long-term maintenance statistics associated with this surgery, it remains somewhat controversial, and some surgeons say the risk of malnutrition or other complications is too great; however, for some patients it can truly be the best option. It almost always cures diabetes, and it is a good choice for some of the highest BMI patients.

If you choose the have a duodenal switch operation, it is imperative to educate yourself on the necessary lifestyle changes and vitamin regimes required. Many duodenal switch patients take 20 or more vitamins a day, and the vitamin regimen must be specific to what you can absorb. The duodenal switch diet is typically very high protein, moderate fat, and low carbohydrate. Simple carbohydrates are still fully absorbed, so even with this powerful operation, patients do not have carte blanche at the dinner table.

What are the risks of the duodenal switch?

Every weight loss surgery has the potential for complications, some extremely serious. The following is a list of potential complications from the duodenal switch, but it isn't an exhaustive list. It's important to talk to your surgeon about potential complications and the probability of these risks in your particular case.

Duodenal switch patients need to be especially well educated about their procedure and their revised anatomy. As this surgery isn't very common, it is vital that patients can accurately explain their anatomy to medical professionals. Patients also need to be educated on what is needed to live a healthy life—what blood tests need to be done regularly, what types of vitamins to take, and so on.

Immediate Surgery Risks:
- Severe bleeding
- Complications of anesthesia
- Infections
- Respiratory problems
- Blood clots
- Gastrointestinal leaks
- Death (rare)

Long Term Risks:
- Bowel obstruction
- Gallstones
- Vomiting
- Hernia

- Malnutrition, vitamin deficiencies
- Ulcers
- Death (rare)

CHAPTER 3
WHY DID YOU CHOOSE THE SLEEVE?

In my experience, one of the most common dilemmas for people is deciding which surgery to choose between gastric bypass and sleeve. It is important to say that there is no single best surgery for everyone. Everyone has different medical circumstances and different life situations that must be considered on an individual basis. Still, it can sometimes be helpful to understand how someone arrives at his or her own conclusions.

Why did you choose the sleeve instead of gastric bypass?

(1) I did not want to dump. Some people see "dumping" as a benefit to the gastric bypass. It trains them to stay away from sugar. When gastric bypass patients eat a high carbohydrate food (often simple carbs) they sometimes

33

become very ill. They may experience nausea, sweating, diarrhea, vomiting, and a general feeling of malaise. I decided that I didn't want to spend the rest of my life in fear of dumping. I'd rather have the freedom to eat whatever kind of food I would like, and I trusted myself to make healthy choices (most of the time). So if I want to taste my young daughter's very first homemade chocolate chip cookie, I can. Like anyone losing weight, I need to account for every calorie, carb, and fat gram….and I don't have to worry about becoming ill if I eat something with sugar. Some gastric bypass patients describe the way they eat as "like a diabetic." Ironically, many of them had the gastric bypass to have freedom from diabetes, but they find they still need to follow the diabetic diet for the rest of their lives in order to avoid dumping syndrome.

(2) I did not want to worry about vitamin malabsorption. I've been slightly anemic for many years. I didn't want a surgery that would be working against me in trying to keep my anemia in check. I also didn't like the idea of having to take an extensive number of vitamins everyday; however, I should point that that I *do* have to take daily vitamins with the sleeve! The difference is, I'm far less likely to have any problems with vitamin deficiency with the sleeve than with any type of intestinal bypass surgery.

(3) I didn't want a "pouch" for a stomach. While it's theoretically possible that the sleeve can stretch, it is believed that the pouch can stretch more. This has to do with the portion of the original stomach that is used to make the new stomach. With the pouch, it includes more of the stretchy greater curvature. With the sleeve, the greater curvature is removed and what is left is more muscular and stretches less.

I also wanted to keep my natural pyloric valve. The pyloric valve regulates food and liquid that goes from the stomach into the small intestines. It ensures that food doesn't go through too quickly, which helps us to remain full. It also isn't prone to causing food to get "stuck." Both of these issues can arise with the pouch of the gastric bypass.

(4) I didn't want a blind stomach. With the gastric bypass, the pouch is separated from the rest of the stomach, and the remaining stomach is sealed up and remains in your body. It is attached to your intestines and continues to produce gastric juices to aid in digestion. Normally, this isn't an issue. In fact, it could be seen as an advantage if it becomes necessary to re-attach the natural stomach to un-do the operation. (Note that while this is possible, it is very complicated and often dangerous. It is very rarely done.) So what is the problem with having a blind stomach? It can still get ulcers, stomach cancer, or other ailments. Normally, when we have an ulcer, the doctor can use a

scope to get into our stomach and look around and even do some repairs. With a blind stomach, however, it cannot be scoped. One would have to have an operation in order for a doctor to access the blind stomach.

Why did you choose the sleeve instead of duodenal switch?

Many of my complaints about the gastric bypass are not issues with the duodenal switch. Here are some reasons I chose the sleeve instead of the duodenal switch.

(1) There were no surgeons in my area, and my insurance wouldn't cover it. In 2008, when I began to seriously research weight loss surgery, the duodenal switch was only offered by one surgeon in my entire state, and he was a four hour drive away. I knew that I wanted a surgeon closer to home so that I can easily go in for follow-up visits and also be active in the surgeon's support group. My insurance company, at the time, would not approve duodenal switch surgery. The policy has since been changed and the company covers duodenal switch surgery for qualified candidates who have a BMI of 50 or more.

The duodenal switch surgery is a more complicated operation than any of the other bariatric surgeries. It's takes longer to do and requires a great deal of skill to handle the very delicate duodenal tissue. For a laundry list of reasons that are outside the scope of this book, including a controversial notion that the surgery is "too risky," the duodenal switch is not widely offered.

(2) I didn't want to take a massive vitamin regimen. Just as gastric bypass patients must take a lot of vitamins, duodenal switch patients must do so as well. In fact, from speaking to duodenal switch patients, it seems that they take even more vitamins than RNY patients. Not only are there a lot of daily pills to take, the rules are also complicated. A, D, E, and K (all fat soluble vitamins) must be taken in dry form. You should take iron with vitamin C. You should take calcium with vitamin D. Iron, zinc, and calcium all must be taken at separate times. Depending on their labs, duodenal switch patients can end up taking a small handful of pills six times a day— for the rest of their lives.

Now, most patients who have had the duodenal switch seem very happy with it and say their vitamin regimen isn't that big a deal. It becomes a habit for them, as easy as brushing their teeth. Certainly, it's a small price to pay for being thin and healthy, but for me, taking all those vitamins fell into the "con" list.

(3) The duodenal switch diet didn't appeal to me. Many patients see the duodenal switch diet as a big plus. As a lifelong vegetarian, I didn't! Most duodenal switch patients eat a lot of protein and a moderate amount of fat. The

duodenal switch community often jokes about their love for bacon. Because their bodies do not absorb much fat, they must eat a good amount of it in order to get enough fat to be healthy. This is a notion that appeals to many people who enjoy high fat and meaty foods, but not to me.

(4) I didn't want a more complicated and involved operation. The sleeve operation took approximately an hour. A duodenal switch operation can take 3 hours and often longer if there are adhesions or other unexpected surprises to slow the surgery down. As more things are cut and altered, there is also more risk for complications.

While the weight loss statistics for the RNY and DS were promising, I just didn't want to have intestinal re-routing. I wanted something that was less invasive and had less potential for long-term complications.

Why did you choose the sleeve instead of the adjustable band?

(1) I didn't like the idea of a "foreign body" in me. For many people, maybe even most people, this may seem trivial. Perhaps it is, but for me, I did not like the idea of having something implanted in my body, something that wasn't supposed to be there. While this alone wasn't enough reason for me to cross the adjustable gastric band off my list, it was part of my thought process.

(2) I had heard too many "stories" about bands slipping and erosion. I wanted a permanent solution, not one that might send me back to the operating table to un-do or revise the first operation. Many people are successful with the band, but after reading a few too many stories on the Internet about bands behaving badly, I didn't want to risk it.

(3) Statistically, the weight loss results are less impressive. Bands might be great for patients with a lower BMI...but I had over 100 pounds to lose.

(4) I didn't want to have to fill and unfill the band. I wanted good restriction, all the time. While some may see the ability to increase or decrease restriction as a plus, I saw it as a negative. I want good restriction for the rest of my life. I've eaten enough big meals. I don't need any more!

For me, the sleeve surgery was the obvious choice. It would give me consistent restriction and would reduce my hunger. There wouldn't be any foreign objects in my body, and I wouldn't have to worry (too much) about vitamin deficiencies or getting ill if I ate the wrong kind of food.

CHAPTER 4
HOW DO YOU HANDLE THE STIGMA OF WEIGHT LOSS SURGERY?

Once I decided to have weight loss surgery, and once I discovered the *right kind* of weight loss surgery for me, I was excited. The sleeve seemed like a light at the end of the tunnel. It seemed as if I finally had a real chance of losing weight and keeping it off. I was thrilled. I was hopeful. I couldn't wait to have the most powerful tool I'd ever used for weight loss on my side.

Not everyone shares this perspective. Some people think weight loss surgery is too extreme. Some think it's the "easy way out." If you decide to have weight loss surgery, you need to know that there is a good chance you will encounter someone who doesn't think the sleeve is as great as you do. I think it is best to just be prepared for this possibility, and think about how you will respond ahead of time.

I've been very fortunate in this regard. The truth is, my family and friends have all be extremely supportive. Everyone understood why I chose to get weight loss surgery. Everyone seemed to trust my own research and my decision. Everyone supported me. The only negative comments I heard were stories from other weight loss surgery patients, and the occasional passing acquaintance. Still, I know this is an issue that very much affects a lot of weight loss surgery patients, so I wanted to address it. It's up to you how open you want to be about your weight loss surgery. Even if you choose to be open, you do not owe anyone an explanation for why you have chosen this path for yourself.

How do you deal with people telling you "I know someone who died after weight loss surgery"?

It must be human nature, but when you let people know you are planning to have weight loss surgery, horror stories seem to come out of the woodwork. I remember when I was pregnant. I heard more horror stories about childbirth the 9 months I was pregnant than I ever had before. It might just be the way some people show concern. Don't be surprised if it seems like almost everyone knows somebody with a bad outcome to a weight loss surgery—even if it's a second cousin's former roommate's mother's friend from high school.

Keep in mind, usually these horror stories are not specific to the sleeve surgery. The sleeve just hasn't been around long enough to generate too many horror stories. Also, many of these stories date back several years. People tend to lump all weight loss surgeries together. Antiqued procedures such as "stomach stapling" and the long-discontinued and risky jejunoileal bypass are not differentiated from safe and more successful modern operations. Weight loss surgery techniques have improved greatly in the last decade. For example, "open" operations used to be done rather than less invasive laparoscopic ones. The risk is far less than it used to be.

Make no mistake, the sleeve is a major operation with very serious risks. Don't let anecdotes scare you away, though. Instead, look at the real statistics for your surgeon's complication and mortality rates, and then make an informed decision on whether or not the surgery is worth the risk. For me, I came to believe that the risks associated with morbid obesity were much higher than the risks associated with sleeve surgery.

How do you respond when people ask "Don't people lose weight and then just gain it all back?"

Skepticism over the likely success of your planned weight loss surgery is understandable. After all, there are some celebrity weight loss surgery patients who did just that. People who haven't looked closely at recent studies, however, may not realize that the sleeve surgery significantly increases your chances of not just losing weight, but keeping it off.

Once a person becomes morbidly obese, the body changes on a hormonal and chemical level. The person's body works to keep the weight on. We evolved to hold on to excess body fat to help us survive in times of famine. Our bodies don't know that most of us living in Western society face very little risk of food scarcity.

Additionally, obese people often develop comorbidities that can actually make weight loss more difficult. Insulin resistance, diabetes, hypothyroid, growth hormone deficiencies, and other medical issues can encourage our bodies to stay fat. Morbidly obese people also sometimes develop mobility issues, which makes exercise difficult. Decreased daily movement has obvious effects on our ability to burn calories.

Once a person becomes morbidly obese, it is increasingly difficult to achieve and maintain significant weight loss. It is estimated that as few as 2% of morbidly obese people who embark on a diet and exercise program lose weight and keep it off (Wing, & Phelan, 2005. Science-based solutions to obesity: What are the roles of academia, government, industry, and health care? *American Journal of Clinical Nutrition* **82**(1), 207S–273S.) With sleeve surgery, one's chance for success is significantly higher than 2%!

How do you respond when people ask "Isn't weight loss surgery a bit extreme?"

I agree with them that weight loss surgery *is* extreme. It is not a decision to be made lightly, and it is life altering. If you explain the operation to someone as a voluntary removal of 75-90% of your stomach, "extreme" is an apt description. For people that get hung up on the idea that weight loss surgery is too extreme, you can gently remind them that morbid obesity is also extreme. Our bodies are not meant to carry around 100 or more extra pounds! This extreme measure to resolve morbid obesity is, in fact, the *most effective* measure.

How do you respond when people ask "Why can't you just diet and exercise?"

For most people who get to the point that they require weight loss surgery in order to regain their health, the suggestion that they should simply try diet and exercise is laughable. *Of course* we have tried diet and exercise, for many, many years. In fact, weight loss surgery programs *require* that patients have tried and failed at diet and exercise measures to control their obesity. Many insurance companies require documentation of 6 months to a full year of a formal diet and exercise program before they will approve the surgery.

When this concern is raised, I like to point out that once a person becomes morbidly obese he or she is very unlikely to be successful in losing and keeping off a substantial amount of weight with diet and exercise alone. Many of us have dieted and exercised our way right up the scale and into the morbidly obese range! Also, once one has weight loss surgery, it isn't a free ticket to weight loss. We have to be very careful about everything we eat for the rest of our lives to ensure adequate nutrition. The most successful losers make exercise part of their everyday lives. We still must diet and exercise to be healthy, but we have a powerful tool that helps increase the odds that *this time* we will lose the weight and keep it off.

How do you respond when people say "you are taking the easy way out"?

First, weight loss surgery is not easy. Yes, it is *easier* to be successful when you have weight loss surgery as a tool, but *easier* does not equal easy. With the risk and pain of surgery, the expense, the lifestyle changes, the tough pre-op diet, the exercise regimens, the support groups, nutritionists, and therapists, it isn't easy; it's a lot of work. It is, however, easier for a morbidly obese person to lose weight and keep it off with weight loss surgery rather than without; however this hardly qualifies it as an "easy way out"!

When it is suggested that weight loss surgery is the "easy way out," the undertone of the message is often that it is somehow morally superior to lose weight with diet and exercise alone rather than with surgery. I cannot understand this. Setting aside for a minute the fact that there is nothing "easy" about weight loss surgery, why is choosing to do something the "easy way" inferior to doing something the "hard way"? I drive my car. I use a microwave. I use a hairdryer. In the winter, I even turn on the furnace at my house rather than building a fire. We all do things the "easy" way when technology allows us to be more efficient. Why is this OK in other aspects of life, but not OK with weight loss?

So when someone says that weight loss surgery is the "easy way out," just smile and tell them it's the *efficient and effective* way. Then, ask the person if he or she use a washing machine or still beats his or her clothes with a rock down by the river. If the person criticizing you uses modern conveniences that make life safer, easier, and more efficient, then he or she is hardly in a position to criticize.

CHAPTER 5
HOW DO I CHOOSE A SURGEON?

Once you've decided that you want to have sleeve surgery, it is important that you find a surgeon who is a good fit. This can be an overwhelming task if you live in a large metropolitan area with a lot of options or live in a more rural area and must commit to traveling.

How do I begin looking for sleeve surgeon?

You can begin by looking into your best local hospitals and learning if they a bariatric program. Additionally, I recommend that you go to the website for the American Society for Metabolic and Bariatric Surgery at www.asmbs.org to search for surgeons in your area. Go to "find a member" under the section "Patients and Public" to do your search.

Not all bariatric surgeons perform sleeve surgeries. Many only do gastric bypass and/or adjustable bands. If you are committed to getting a sleeve surgery, it is important that you go to a surgeon who performs sleeve surgeries. That might seem like a rather obvious statement, but many patients have been known to go to a surgeon who only does gastric bypass and adjustable bands and find that they get a sales pitch for why they should do a different surgery.

More and more surgeons are performing sleeve surgeries; however, many still cling to the long-running "gold standard" surgery—the gastric bypass. Do not waste your time going to a surgeon who doesn't offer the surgery in which you are interested. Many surgeons list the procedures offered on their websites, or you can find out by calling their office. I recommend that you do this before you even attend an information session (which is usually the first step in becoming a patient).

If your health insurance covers bariatric surgery, you will want to check with your insurance company to find out what surgeons are in the network. Often, insurance companies require surgeons to be working at a designated "Center of Excellence" in order to approve benefits. Your insurance company should be able to provide you with a list of eligible surgeons in your area.

What sort of statistics should I look for in a surgeon?

Surgeons keep track of complication and mortality rates. Mortality rates show how many patients died during or shortly after surgery. Complication rates show how many patients had complications during or shortly after surgery. As you know, there is a laundry list of possible complications from surgery. So when I was looking for a sleeve surgeon, I focused on two statistics that I believed were especially important: death rate and leak rate.

The death rate, obviously, is important. You need to know what percentage of this surgeon's patients died while under his or her care. Ideally, of course, you want a 0% death rate; however, even the very best surgeons in the country sometimes lose a patient. In fact, sometimes the best surgeons have a slightly *higher* death rate because they are willing to take on very high risk patients that other surgeons will not touch. Also, some surgeons with a 0% death rate simply do not perform a large number of bariatric surgeries so they have a small sample size and have just "gotten lucky" so far. Because of these issues, the death rate, in itself, doesn't tell the whole story...but it is a starting point.

Leaks are more common with the sleeve than with gastric bypass or adjustable gastric banding. A leak happens when a small amount of gastric juices from the stomach is excreted into the body. This can be an easy fix or a life-threatening situation. Because the sleeve has a very long staple line where the stomach is removed, the risk of leaks is higher than with the gastric bypass where the staple line is much shorter.

According to the Updated Position Statement on Sleeve Gastrectomy as a Bariatric Procedure from the American Society for Metabolic and Bariatric Surgery in October 2011, staple line leaks and bleeding are the two most serious complications of the sleeve surgery, and these occur at a rate of 1-3%. If a surgeon has a higher leak rate than average, you may want to look for another surgeon.

Does it matter if a surgeon is far away from where I live?

For some patients, traveling to see a surgeon is the only option. If you live in a more rural area, there may not be any sleeve surgeons in your area. Some surgeons, particularly those who perform the duodenal switch surgery, are used to accommodating travelers. Look on their website or call their office to see if they have advice and information for out-of-town patients. They may be able to offer you information on local hotels where they want you to stay after your surgery.

Other patients find they need to travel for a surgeon due to costs. If a patient doesn't have insurance that covers sleeve surgery, the patient may need to find a surgeon that offers a "self pay" option. The cost of a self-pay sleeve in the US can range anywhere from less than $15,000 to well over $25,000. Some patients travel out of the country in search of a "better deal." Such a practice is well outside of my experience and expertise, so I will not comment on this option other than to encourage you to approach it only as an option with *extreme* caution and much research.

A few downsides of having to travel to see a surgeon include follow-up visits and support. Most surgeons want to see their patients at regular intervals after surgery. This is to ensure you are healing properly and that you are sticking to the program. If you have the time and money to travel to these appointments, that is ideal. Some surgeons, especially those who are accustomed to accommodating travelers, can make arrangements with your primary care doctor for follow-up visits.

Most surgeons' offices are staffed with counselors, nutritionists, support groups, and even personal trainers to help lead you down the road to success. If your surgeon is across the country, it will be hard for you to take advantage of these resources. It will be important that you build your own local support team. See a local counselor if you need to work on emotional eating issues. Utilize an online support group, and hire your own personal trainer. For the most part, the conveniences of having a local surgeon can be easily overcome if you are willing to work hard and organize your own team of professional and personal support.

For most patients, having a surgeon in easy driving distance from your home is best; however, take heart if this is not an option. Find the very best surgeon you can and travel to see him or her and also invest in piecing together a good support system closer to home.

What sort of questions should I ask a surgeon and his staff before deciding?

Different surgeon's offices will have different procedures for how new patients are handled. Some surgeons and their staff won't even talk to potential patients until these individuals attend an information session or seminar. If this is the case, sign up for a seminar and bring your questions there. Other offices will let you schedule an initial consult right away. Sometimes these consults are with the surgeon and sometimes they are with a nurse or other health professional. Ideally, you'll want to meet with the surgeon before you decide which surgeon you will choose to perform your surgery, but in some cases, surgeons do not meet with patient until they've already jumped through many hoops on the way to getting approved for the surgery.

It's a good idea to make a list of questions ahead of time to ensure you don't forget anything. Here are some questions to consider to help you get started:

- Is this a Center of Excellence?
- How long have you been offering the sleeve surgery?
- How many sleeve surgeries have you done in total?
- How many sleeve surgeries do you perform in a month or week?
- Are all of your surgeries preformed laparoscopically?

- What hospital do you use for bariatric surgeries?
- What sort of pre-op testing will you require?
- What requirements do you have for patients to approve surgery beyond what insurance requires?
- Are you able to help me obtain insurance approval?
- Do you have self-pay options?
- Does the program offer dedicated nutritionists?
- Do you offer psychological support services and counseling?
- Do you have an active support group?
- Will you work with my primary care doctor?
- Do you offer plastic surgery services after weight loss?
- Do you offer any special support for out-of-town patients?
- Could you please share your complication and mortality rates?
- What is the average weight loss for your sleeve patients?
- What size do you make the sleeve (bougie size or approximate percentage of stomach removed)?
- If you are not available, is there someone on call if I have complications after I go home from surgery?

What should I ask a potential surgeon about surgical technique?

As the sleeve surgery is still relatively new, there is not yet a fully standardized way in which to do the surgery. Most surgeons use a French bougie (FB)or a scope to help guide the size of the sleeve. The smaller the bougie, the smaller the sleeve. The smaller the sleeve, the more restriction you will have. There is some anecdotal evidence that a smaller sleeve is less likely to stretch over time and may help promote greater weight loss; however, there is also some evidence that sleeves that are "too small" have a greater likelihood for complications such as the stomach twisting or problems with GERD later. Again, as of right now, this is purely anecdotal and no solid studies have come forward to support or deny these popular claims.

When you ask the surgeon what size sleeve he makes, he may tell you the bougie size he uses, but some surgeons don't use a bougie. They may use a scope or other device to help guide the shape of the stomach. They might tell you that they remove a certain percentage of the stomach (such as 85%), or they might tell you that your stomach will hold approximately 2 ounces after surgery.

Similarly, you may want to ask your surgeon how he seals your new stomach shut. Does he use staples? Does he use a combination of staples and stitches? Does he "oversew" the sleeve to help make it even tighter? Good information to know, but this shouldn't necessarily be a deal breaker.

Virtually all sleeve surgeries are done laparoscopically. There may be times, however, when a surgeon needs to convert to an open surgery. Ask your surgeon how many of his surgeries are completed laparoscopically.

Does it matter that different surgeons have different surgical techniques?

Some people give more credence to the bougie size than they should. As long as it is significantly smaller than before surgery, and as long as you follow all the rules of post-op life, you will do just fine. The relatively insignificant differences between a 32 FB and a 36 FB are very unlikely to make a difference in your future success. Just as I've seen people struggle with weight regain with a small bougie, I've seen people keep it off successfully with a larger one. The fact is, all standard bougies commonly used in sleeve surgery (32-40 FB is a popular range) will give you a very small stomach that can help you lose a significant amount of weight.

What sort of support services should I be looking for when choosing a surgeon?

Ideally, you'll want a team of professionals to help you pre-op and post-op. Not all surgeons' offices offer all of these services. It's up to you to decide which ones are the most important to you.

- Psychological services

- Support groups
- Nutritionist and dietitians with experience and training in advising with bariatric patients
- Insurance support – someone dedicated to helping you get your insurance approved
- Personal trainers – especially ones experienced with working with bariatric patients
- Bariatric nurses and/or coordinators readily available to answer your questions when the surgeon is not available

CHAPTER 6
WILL INSURANCE PAY FOR THE SLEEVE?

More and more insurance companies are covering weight loss surgery, and a growing number of those companies are adding the sleeve to the list of approved surgeries. The requirements for getting approval for the sleeve surgery vary from company to company. Typically, the requirements for sleeve surgery are the same as requirements for other bariatric surgeries, such as the gastric bypass. Most insurance companies require that your BMI is 40 or greater or 35 and greater with at least two comorbidities. Many insurance companies require a weight history, documentation proving that you've been morbidly obese for at least 5 years. Many insurance companies require that you have proof of some previous weight loss attempts.

What is the first step in finding out if the sleeve is covered by insurance?

The first step is contacting your insurance company. You should have documentation showing what is covered. Some companies offer this documentation online. If you call your insurance company, be sure to take note of the person you speak with in case you need to refer back to the conversation later. When you call, the person you speak with may not know what a "vertical sleeve gastrectomy" is, so be sure to say that you are interested in learning about the coverage the company offers for bariatric surgery.

Gather as much information as you can in writing about your coverage for bariatric surgery. Once you have this information, you can contact your bariatric coordinator or insurance specialist at the office of your surgeon-of-choice. The coordinator can often help walk you through the steps you need in order to obtain approval. Often, these experts are familiar with various insurance companies and will know how easy or difficult the company is to work with. Bariatric coordinators are also experts at reading the fine print and can help you avoid any loopholes in your coverage that could result in a denial.

Will any sort of weight loss program qualify for the required 6-month (or 3-month, or 1-year) diet?

This answer to this really depends on your insurance company. Many insurance companies that specify a pre-op weight loss program list the requirements of these weight loss programs. Usually, the programs must be medically supervised. Sometimes the insurance company specifies what that means—such as monthly weigh-ins with the doctor. Sometimes the company requires evidence of nutritional counseling and exercise. Some insurance companies will accept programs like Weight Watches, some will not. Often this diet program must have been completed within five years, or even one year, prior to weight loss surgery. One thing that insurance companies have in common is that virtually all that require a pre-op diet also require documentation.

Documentation could be medical records from your primary care doctor's office, receipts from paying for a diet meal service plan, evidence of membership to Weight Watchers, etc. Your insurance company or your insurance coordinator will advise you on what sort of documentation you may need.

Many patients who choose to have bariatric surgery have a long history of dieting on their own, but their dieting efforts do not meet the strict criteria of the insurance company. For this reason, it is common for bariatric surgeons to offer (or refer patients to) a medically supervised weight loss program that *does* meet insurance requirements. These programs can be 3 months, 6 months, or a year in length depending on the requirements of your particular insurance company. While participating in a program, you will be placed on a medically supervised diet and offered nutrition counseling. Some insurance companies require evidence of support group participation, and you will be asked to start attending support groups right away. Whatever your insurance company requires for a pre-op diet, most surgeons' offices will be able to help you meet those requirements.

What should I do if my request is denied?

An insurance denial is not the end of the road, but it can be a major bump. If your surgeon's office has an insurance coordinator, he or she will likely work with you to try to appeal. You will need to do some legwork too, but with the expert guidance of the coordinator you can improve your odds of getting approval.

If you have been denied, you should be given a specific reason for why you were denied. Perhaps the company representative didn't see evidence of participation in a support group. Perhaps there was something missing from your diet program, such as a missed weigh-in, and you'll need to complete another month.

If your insurance company covers bariatric surgery, you medically qualify for weight loss surgery, *and* you are seeing an approved weight loss surgeon, most denials can be sorted out. It may feel like everything is moving at a glacial pace but don't give up. It will be well worth your efforts.

Are there options if I don't have insurance or if my insurance doesn't cover the sleeve?

Yes, there are options. Many surgeons offer a self-pay option. They may require that you pay all at once or you may be able to work out an installment payment plan. Self-pay can cost varies greatly by region. You can expect to pay anywhere from less than $15,000 to $25,000 or more.

If you have insurance, but the company just doesn't cover bariatric surgery or the sleeve, you may want to ask the insurance agent if the company would cover the costs of any complications you might have from the surgery. If not, there are insurance policies that you can purchase to cover complications that occur with bariatric surgery. Even though most surgeries are complication-free, when they do occur they can be extremely costly. Speak to your surgeon's office for more information on this. Some surgeons help patients obtain this special insurance.

CHAPTER 7
WHAT IS THE PRE-OP DIET?

Once your insurance has pre-approved your surgery
and you have met all the criteria of your surgeon to
move forward with the surgery, you will still have at
least one final task before your surgery day—the pre-op
diet. By pre-op diet, I don't mean the 6-month
medically supervised diet that your insurance company
required. Most, but not all, surgeons require a final
(and mercifully brief!) pre-op diet right before surgery.
Many weight loss surgery patients say that the pre-op
diet is the hardest part of the entire process!

**How long will I need to diet before the sleeve
operation?**

This is entirely at the discretion of your surgeon.
For surgeons who require pre-op diet, they typically

have a standard diet that all patients must follow. For some, it is a 2-week liquid diet. Others only need to diet for a week and are allowed some solid foods. One thing that most pre-op diets have in common is that they use protein shakes and they are high protein, low carbohydrate, low calorie diets.

What does a typical pre-op diet look like?

A liquid diet seems to be the most popular pre-op diet. Often, patients will have 4-5 small protein shakes a day, plenty of water, and not much else. My surgeon was a bit more liberal in what he allowed. I had 3 protein shakes a day *or* 4 sugar-free instant breakfasts drinks a day. The protein shakes were ones that the surgeon recommended and sold through his office, although they could also be purchased online or at some health food stores. The taste took some getting used to, to be honest. I found that if I froze the shakes, not rock-solid but to a thick slushy consistency, it made them more palatable. In addition, I was allowed to have clear liquids as long as they were sugar free and not carbonated. Examples included sugar free lemonade, sugar free gelatin, and vegetable broth. I was also allowed up to about 150 calories worth of "real food" as long as that food was on a pre-approved list that consisted of mostly vegetables. The food that I would eat on a typical day on the pre-op diet was 3 protein shakes plus a small salad (no dressing) or a small bowl of homemade vegetable soup. My average caloric intake while on this diet was approximately 800 calories a day.

Does it matter if I cheat on the pre-op diet?

While the pre-op diet can seem frustratingly strict, there is a reason for it. The commonly cited purpose of the pre-op diet is to shrink the liver.   An enlarged and fatty liver is difficult to operate around, and there is an increased chance of the liver getting in the way or getting nicked during surgery. Many surgeons go so far as to say that they can *tell* if a patient has cheated on the pre-op diet the moment they see the liver. My nurse told me that she knew of a patient who cheated on the pre-op diet; the surgeon saw the liver, and sewed the patient back up without doing the surgery.

To be honest, I am not sure if stories like this are entirely true or if they are exaggerated and meant as a scare tactic to keep patients "honest." In any case, it is important to be compliant with your pre-op diet. If your surgeon requires it, you should follow the pre-op diet as precisely as humanly possible. If you make a mistake, let the surgeon's office know, and then leave it up to the surgeon to decide if he or she needs to move your surgery date as a result.

Pre-op diets are not without controversy. There are indeed surgeons who do not require a pre-op diet. They say a pre-op diet does NOT decrease the risk of surgical complications and they see no purpose in it. Their patients will typically need to do a liquid diet for 12-24 hours before surgery as is recommended for all types of abdominal surgeries. They will not, however, have to suffer through two weeks of chalky protein shakes.

Regardless of whether you believe a pre-op diet is a good idea or not, if your surgeon recommends one, you should follow it closely. Think of it this way—you are about to alter the way you eat for the rest of your life. After surgery, you *must* comply with post-op diet rules or you risk seriously hurting yourself. If you can be compliant on a strict pre-op diet, you will find your post-op diet a breeze. Yes, your diet will still be strict, but you'll have the benefit of your new weight loss tool to help you! Think of it as your "last diet" without the benefit of sleeve support, and make yourself proud by adhering to it exactly as your surgeon outlines!

Can I use any kind of protein shake for my pre-op diet?

You might have the flexibility of using any kind of protein shake that you wish, or your surgeon may want you to use a specific shake. As previously stated, it is important to follow whatever instructions your surgeon's office provides you. If you do have the flexibility to use any kind of protein shake that you wish, this is a great time to try out a few different brands. Most people have pretty strong opinions about which protein shakes are most palatable, but rarely agree with each other! So it's important to experiment with different kinds. Ideally, try to buy samples of shakes rather than an entire jug of protein shake mix.

If you find one terrible, you'd hate to be stuck with the entire jug!

You can experiment a bit with the shakes, but make sure it's always within the parameters of your pre-op diet plan. Try freezing the shakes, or blending them with ice, to change their consistency. Try adding a bit more or less water than the instructions require. This won't change the total calorie count, but it will change the taste and texture a bit. You might find you like your shakes a bit thicker or thinner than the standard instructions indicate. If your pre-op diet allows you to eat some fruit, try blending your shake with some fruit for extra flavor and a thicker texture. Bananas are great for this! If you use frozen fruit, such as frozen strawberries, you'll find the texture is much thicker and more like a frozen ice cream shake than if you blend with fresh strawberries. Rather than using water, some people like to add the shake mix and some ice cubes to coffee (if the plan allows) and create a sweet iced mocha drink, or they use a vanilla shake mix as a creamer in their coffee. Experiment, and you'll find some combinations that you like!

Many patients, me included, find that their tastes change after surgery. A shake that you liked before surgery may not taste too good after surgery! Again, don't buy in bulk! Wait until after your surgery and you are cleared for full liquids, and then buy single servings whenever possible to test different brands and flavors.

CHAPTER 8
WHAT IS SURGERY DAY LIKE?

Your day is finally here! You've passed all the required steps and you feel confident and ready to start your new life. While you may feel confident in your decision about surgery, don't be surprised if you are very nervous too. This is a major life changing surgery with serious risks. Being a little nervous is a good sign that you understand that; however, if you are more than just a little nervous and you have serious doubts...talk to your surgeon! If you have unanswered questions or if you still are very uncertain that this is the right thing for you to do, you can still cancel your procedure. My surgeon liked to say that you can change your mind up until the point that they knock you out!

Most patients who get to the point of having a surgery date for their sleeve operation are reasonably ready. Many research surgeries for years before finally deciding it is right for them. Most patients have to jump through many hoops just to get a date on the calendar, so they have had plenty of time to consider their decision from all angles.

Although it might be a challenge, do everything you can to get a good night's sleep before your surgery. Your surgeon will likely have you on clear liquids only for the day before surgery and then nothing by mouth after 10 pm or midnight the night before surgery. These instructions do vary a bit, so be sure to follow the orders your surgeon gives you. If you have any questions about preparing for the surgery, ask!

What do I need to do the day before surgery?

The day before surgery you will likely be on clear liquids. Yes, this can be a challenge and you will likely be pretty hungry, but, most patients find they are so nervous and excited about the surgery that it really isn't too bad. My surgeon allowed broth and gelatin the day before surgery. In fact, he even allowed full-sugar gelatin to give some extra calories the day before surgery. My calorie count for the day, though, was well under 500.

Be sure to ask your surgeon what prescription medications you should continue to take the day before surgery. There are some medications that your surgeon may want you to stop the day before, or even a few days before, surgery.

The day before surgery I made my final preparations. My bag was packed, my childcare was verified, and my prayer requests were sent out! I tried to get a good night's sleep, but to be honest I only slept for about 3 hours that night. I was anxious to get to the hospital early the next morning and start my big journey!

What should I bring with me to the hospital?

You don't need to bring too much. Ask your surgeon's office staff for the protocol, but most often sleeve surgeries are done with just a one-night stay in the hospital. If this is the case, you will just need your standard toiletries (toothbrush, deodorant, etc.) plus a change of clothes. The clothes you pack to go home in should be very loose fitting and comfortable. You definitely don't want anything that will be tight around your abdomen. A loose old pair of sweatpants is a good solution. I also highly recommend that you pack some good quality lip moisturizer. You won't be allowed to eat or drink for a while after surgery, and lip moisturizer can make a difference in how comfortable you feel!

You will likely spend a lot of time resting after the surgery, so you may want to bring a favorite book or magazine. Most hospitals have TVs in the room, but you may also want to bring a laptop or tablet computer to keep yourself entertained.

Should I bring someone with me to the hospital?

You will definitely need someone to drive you home from the hospital. It's also beneficial to have someone with you to be your advocate. A good friend or spouse can help make sure the nurses know if you need another dose of pain medication! Plus, they can help you as you start taking short walks around the hospital floor to minimize the risk of blood clots.

How long will the surgery take?

This varies a lot by surgeon and by any complications that may be encountered during the surgery. My surgery was completed in less than an hour. Sometimes, however, the surgery can take two hours or more. You can ask your surgeon ahead of time how long the sleeve surgery typically takes him or her to complete.

Will I be in a lot of pain when I wake up?

I've had a couple of surgeries in my life, and I can tell you that I *always* seem to wake up moaning and asking for pain medicine. With the sleeve surgery, when I woke up I did feel some pain, and I could hear myself moaning before I was even fully awake. Honestly, I sounded much worse than I felt.

A nurse told me that some patients wake up peacefully, some moaning, and some wake with a scream and usually it has nothing to do with the pain level they are experiencing. It's simply a reaction to coming out of anesthesia. If you want to hear some interesting stories, talk to recovery room nurses! Don't worry, no matter how you react in those moments when you wake up from anesthesia, you will not surprise them. They've seen it all!

The pain itself was quite manageable when I woke up. I was still very groggy and out of it from surgery, and whatever pain medicine they had given me had masked most of the pain. The pain that *was* still there, I was too out-of-it to really care much about. I was in a recovery room with many other patients, separated by curtains. Some patients were moaning, but it was mostly pretty quiet. A nurse was at my side moments after I opened my eyes.

The surgery will literally seem like a blink of your eyes. You will be wheeled into the O.R. The hospital personnel might ask you to help move your body from the bed you were wheeled in on to the operating table. The anesthesiologist will then talk you through what he or she is doing, and the next thing you know you are waking up in the recovery room!

Will they use a catheter?

It depends. Some surgeons use a urinary catheter as part of normal protocol, and some do not. My surgeon did not because the surgery was so short, and he also wanted to encourage his sleeve patients to get up and start walking soon after the procedure. If your surgeon does require a catheter, it is typically inserted after you are already under anesthesia. Sometimes it is removed before you wake up, so you'd never know you had one unless you were told. More often, though, the nurses will leave it in for a few hours after you wake up. This allows you to stay in bed and rest rather than having to get up and use the restroom if you need to urinate. Some surgeons also like to closely monitor urine output after surgery, which can easily be accomplished with a catheter. A nurse will remove the catheter, which can feel a bit funny but isn't usually painful.

Will I have a drain?

This is also a good question to ask your surgeon ahead of time. Some surgeons use a drain, some do not. Of the surgeons who do use a drain, some will remove it before you leave the hospital, and some will require that you return to their office to have it removed.

I had a drain, called a "JP drain." It looked like a clear plastic grenade coming out of my left side (called the "bulb"), attached to some tubing. Red liquid, which eventually became light pink slowly filled the bulb. The surgeon gave me instructions for clearing the drain and keeping the site clean. I used a safety pin to attach it to the top of my pants, so that it wouldn't dangle or get in the way. I had my drain in for a week after surgery.

A week after surgery, I went to the surgeon's office for a check-up and the nurse removed my drain. I will tell you, it was a very strange sensation to have the drain removed! It didn't hurt, it was just…strange. The nurse pulled the tubing out, and I was surprised to see how much tubing had been inside of me! It was a relief to have it removed and it felt like a big milestone in my recovery.

How soon after surgery will I be able to eat or drink?

This varies by hospital and surgeon. Are you noticing a trend here? Most details of the sleeve surgery vary by surgeon! You will be on IV fluids, so you shouldn't have to worry about become too dehydrated. You may find that your lips become very parched, and your throat becomes very dry. If you didn't bring your own, ask a nurse for some lip balm. A lot of hospitals will also offer you a tiny sponge on a stick to help wet the inside of your mouth.

Most surgeons won't let you eat or drink anything until you've had a leak test. For a leak test, you will likely be transported from your hospital room to the radiology department. You will be asked to stand on a platform in front of a large machine and drink a small amount of thin barium. The radiologist will watch the barium go through your stomach and ensure there are no leaks. If you pass the leak test, you will be allowed to drink for the first time!

The first time I was allowed to drink a sip of water, I was very nervous. I took the sip very slowly, not knowing how my newly sleeved stomach would react. Fortunately, it went down just fine. It is important to be very slow and cautious, though, the first time you take a sip of water!

What happens if I don't pass the leak test?

The answer to this really depends on the extent of the leak. Small leaks sometimes do not require another surgery, but you will likely need an extended hospital stay (and IV nutrient support) until it heals. Some leaks require an operation to go back in and fix the problem. While leaks are rare, they are more common with the sleeve surgery than then gastric bypass because of the length of the staple line. There is just more area to potentially develop a leak!

If I pass the leak test, does that mean I'm in the clear for leaks?

No, it just means that you don't have an apparent leak at the time of the test. Leaks can develop up to several weeks after the surgery if too much stress is put on the stomach. This is why it is so crucial to follow your surgeon's post-op dietary plan precisely. Sometimes, even if you follow all the rules, you can still develop a leak. It could be that a small leak was present since the time of surgery, but it just didn't grow large enough to show itself until later.

What will I be allowed to eat?

Your first "food" will look similar to what you were allowed to eat the day before surgery—clear liquids. My first meal was apple juice and jello. You must sip very, very slowly. Anything more than a small sip can be painful. You new tiny little stomach is swollen and cannot hold much, and you don't want to put any pressure on the fresh staple lines. Err on the side of caution when it comes to how much you eat and drink. The most important thing is staying hydrated, and while you are in the hospital, you are on IV fluids to assist with this!

What will I be doing after surgery while I'm in the hospital?

Your nurses will start pushing you to walk pretty much from the moment they move you from the recovery room to your hospital room. The sooner you start moving, the better. At first, it will take a long time to just walk from your bed to the bathroom. You'll need help, especially to make sure you are stable and don't fall. Before the day is over, however, you will likely be walking laps around the hospital floor, dragging along your IV pole with you. Walking frequently not only minimizes the risks of blood clots, it also helps you feel better faster. It will help get the anesthesia out of your system and get your heart pumping so that you can heal faster.

Once you pass the leak test, you can add sipping to your list of activities. You won't be allowed to use a straw as they don't want you to swallow any air. You'll spend your remaining time in the hospital sipping, walking, resting, sipping, walking, resting, and so on!

How much pain will I have after I leave the hospital?

Some sleevers leave the hospital with very little discomfort. Many say they never needed the prescription pain medications they were sent home with from their surgeon. Others require the prescription pain medication for a week or even two weeks. How you will feel after surgery really depends on many factors. Pre-existing medical conditions that slow healing or surgical complications will affect how you feel after surgery. In addition, the need for pain medication will be affected by how soon and how much you start moving after surgery and your individual tolerance to pain.

For me, the pain lasted for a couple of weeks. At two weeks out, I was still sensitive and when I moved in certain ways I would still get a sharp pain on my right side. In speaking with my surgeon, he explained that where I felt the pain was right in the area where the muscles were separated so the stomach could be pulled out. He said it was a spot at which many of his sleeve patients experienced lingering pain. It will pass. I had to tell myself this fact over and over again some days— *it will pass*. About two weeks after surgery, it did indeed pass. If you are ever unsure if a pain is normal or not, call your surgeon's office. Don't wonder and worry or wait for it to get worse.

CHAPTER 9
WHAT ARE THE FIRST FEW WEEKS LIKE?

Everyone's recovery is different. The most important thing you can do is follow the instructions of your surgeon precisely. Don't expect to do much more that rest, shuffle around, and sip lots of water for the first few days.

How soon will I be back on my feet?

The answer to this depends on a lot of factors. What medical conditions do you have that might slow your healing? How mobile were you before surgery? How fit were you before surgery? Did you have any complications during surgery or immediately after?

Many people are up and doing light activities as soon as they return home from the hospital. Others might need a week of rest in their favorite recliner before they venture into resuming any normal activities. Regardless of your activity level, there is a bare minimum you need to do in the days and weeks after surgery. Your surgeon can guide you on what an appropriate activity level is for you. For most patients, however, we are advised to walk every other hour.

Patients are advised to sip on lots of water. While your goal for sipping water will ultimately be at least 64 ounces, don't worry if you can only get in 30 or 40 ounces, for example, in those early days. You'll find that you cannot swallow much at a time and you must take a long pause between sips—otherwise your stomach might hurt. As long as you make it a priority to keep sipping, you'll find that you're able to drink more every day. Before you know it, you'll be drinking 64 ounces and even 100 ounces every day without a problem! Remember that all clear liquids "count" towards that goal of 64 ounces. A frozen sugar-free popsicle can be a delicious treat and can be included in your efforts to increase your fluid intake.

The goal in recovery should be progress. Every day, you can walk a little further and sip a little more water. Don't push yourself too hard in either area, or you could have a set back. I found that in the first three weeks of recovery, I had days where I felt pretty good. On some of those days, I overdid it. I would lift something that was a bit too heavy or not be careful enough when I twisted my body and moved. I would get a sharp pain that would send me back to my recliner and set back my recovery. I'd be back to shuffling around the house slowly for the rest of the day. So even when you are feeling better, you must be careful to not overdo things and set back your progress!

Why did I gain weight in the hospital?!

I should have listened to the nurse at the hospital who told me not to weigh myself for at least 2 weeks. I think my mistake was understandable. After all, I had just gone through the pain and risk of a major surgery in order to lose weight—I wanted to know what I weighed! You can imagine how I felt when I stepped on the scale the day after I got home from the hospital, 3 days after my surgery, and saw that I had *gained* 9 pounds! I had eaten almost nothing for the past 3 days and even had most of my stomach removed. How could I gain 9 pounds?

All those IV fluids were the culprit. You are pumped with fluids from the moment you enter the hospital to right before you leave. You aren't able to ingest much by mouth, and the doctors and nurses know that during your first days home from surgery your fluid intake will also be lower than normal, so they pump you up. Also, the shock and stress you body is under from the surgery can cause you to retain more water weight. So, my advice to you is to not get on the scale until at least 2 weeks after surgery. If you must, just do so knowing there is a good chance you have gained weight.

The more you walk and move, the quicker you will lose this weight. Some lose it in a couple of days, some take a couple of weeks. For me, it was a full 7 days after surgery before I got back down to my pre-surgery weight.

What sort of help will I need in the days after surgery?

Most patients are able to make their own meals after surgery when they get home; however do not expect to make meals for the entire family. Your meals will be easy to make—mostly shakes and broths early on—so you will likely feel capable of making them. You also should be fine to use the restroom and shower on your own, but if you feel unsure or shaky, it's good to have someone nearby.

You will not be able to do household chores, especially those that require bending or lifting, for at least a couple of weeks. Chores that do not require lifting or much bending, like light dusting, might be fine. Most chores, though, will need to be put on hold until you heal. This means, you should ask someone else to do the laundry or scrub the floors!

Child care can be difficult, because young kids require a lot of bending, lifting, and other maneuvers that you shouldn't be doing right after major abdominal surgery. It will be important to arrange for child care assistance if you have young children. If your children are toddlers or younger, be sure to have child care assistance in place at least until your lifting restrictions are removed.

So while you will be able to take care of yourself, for the most part, you will not be of much use in taking care of others right after surgery. If you are a stay-at-home parent or your household duties include a lot of heavy lifting, be sure to make arrangements for someone else to help with these roles until you are healed. While you might "feel" like you can do these things much sooner, it is better to err on the side of caution and line up help for at least one or two weeks following your surgery.

Will I be hungry?

While some patients do say they experienced hunger after surgery, I was lucky to fall into the majority here and did not feel any hunger. I ate as required by my schedule, but never because I felt hungry. A reduction in hunger is one of the greatest features of the sleeve surgery, and one of the reasons that it is so successful. Not only will small portions of food fill you up very quickly, but you also won't be very hungry to begin with! This is thanks, in part, to a massive reduction in the hormone ghrelin. Ghrelin is a hormone produced by your stomach (and elsewhere too, but mostly your stomach). It signals your brain that you are hungry. By removing most of the stomach, you are removing a large portion of ghrelin production.

Although the relationship between obesity and ghrelin are still being studied, it is generally believed that having less ghrelin will mean you are less hungry. In fact, there has even been research conducted to try to make an "obesity vaccine" that works by blocking ghrelin (Zorrilla, Iwasaki, Moss, Chang, Otsuji, Inoue, Meijler, & Janda, 2006. Vaccination against weight gain. *Proceedings of the National Academy of Sciences* **103**[35], 13226–31.)

For those patients who do feel hunger, it is possibly due to a lot of stomach acid. A lot of acid in your stomach can mimic the feelings of hunger. You may want to ask your surgeon about taking an acid reducer to see if it helps minimize your hunger.

What will my diet look like after surgery?

If you've read this far into the book, I bet you can guess what I am going to say here. Your post-op diet will vary depending on what your surgeon recommends. Different surgeons have different plans. Most plans, however, do have a few things in common. They generally start as liquids-only and slowly progress to pureed foods and then soft foods. Eventually, you'll be eating regular consistency. This was my post-op diet plan:

Week 1: Clear liquids (sugar free drinks, no sugar added juice, broth, gelatin)

Week 2-3: Full liquids (protein shakes, strained soups)

Week 4: Pureed foods (yogurt, low fat pudding, foods pureed to a baby food consistency)

Week 5-6: Soft foods (cottage cheese, tofu, soft-cooked meats and eggs)

Week 7 onwards: Regular foods, except raw vegetables or raw fibrous fruit (introduced slowing and carefully)

Month 3 onwards: slow introduction of raw vegetables and raw fruit

While I was only eating an average of 400-500 calories a day for the first few weeks, by week four I was able to get into my targeted weight loss range of 600-800 calories per day. With everything I ate, I had to focus on getting a high enough protein and water in take. Here is a summary of my weight loss diet. Keep in mind that your diet might vary from this and you should stick with whatever plan your nutritionist and surgeon outline for you:

My Daily Sleeve Diet (while in weight loss phase)
Calories: 600-800
Carbs: Less than 60 grams a day (ideally around 40)
Protein: At least 65 grams a day (ideally, around 75)
Water: At least 64 ounces a day (ideally around 80)

Your nutritionist or surgeon will give you guidelines to follow. Some offices give the same guidelines to all patients while others tweak their guidelines to match the needs of every individual patient. Obviously the larger you are and the more muscle mass you have, the more calories you can consume and still lose weight. Also, as you begin to add exercise to your daily routine you might need more calories or more carbohydrates—as well as more water—in order to stay healthy and strong.

Do you have to track all your food in a daily log?

My surgeon did not require this, although I chose to do it. From what I had seen in my support group, weight loss surgery patients who keep detailed records of what they had eaten seemed to be far more successful in meeting their goals then those who did not.

Now, before you roll your eyes and say "That sounds just like another diet," let me assure you that "dieting" with the sleeve is NOTHING like being on another diet. I'm not hungry; I'm not craving sweets; I don't feel like I'm watching the clock desperate for when I can have my next meal or snack. You still enjoy food, but you don't obsess about it. You sometimes will find yourself needing to be *reminded* to eat. You eat because your body needs the fuel. It's as simple as that. It's a completely different experience, and it's very liberating.

By writing down everything you eat, you can be sure that you are accountable. It'll help prevent thoughtless grazing. It will ensure you are getting enough protein. It will help you to tweak your diet when you hit a weight loss stall. If you need some help with your diet, it will give you a record that you can take to your nutritionist.

There are many wonderful online tools you can use to track your daily intake. Many of them are free, and most can even be accessed from your cell phone. I enjoyed (and still use!) Livestrong's The Daily Plate (www.livestrong.com/thedailyplate). It keeps track of everything I eat and the water I drink and helps me track my progress with weight loss and BMI changes and even has a place to chart your changes in measurements.

If you prefer, you can always use a good old-fashioned paper and pencil. Just be sure that you carefully measure and weigh everything you eat—at least while you are in the weight loss phase of your journey. Whenever possible, avoid eyeballing or estimating how much you are eating. The more accurate you can be in your food logs, the more likely you will be successful.

Does this mean I won't be successful if I don't want to keep a food log?

If you don't want to keep a food log, it does not mean you won't be successful. Many people successfully lose weight with the sleeve without counting calories or keeping a log. For some people, the stress or inconvenience of keeping a food log is too much. Patients who choose to not use a food log need to be especially mindful of a few things. First, they must make sure they are only eating a set number of times a day. This might be three meals and two snacks, for example. This will help to minimize any grazing, which can add unwanted calories to your daily intake. Second, patients who don't keep a food log must be certain to always eat protein first at every meal. It is important to eat enough protein, so filling up on carbs before eating the protein is a sure way to increase the risk of a deficiency. Third, they need to keep an eye on the scale. If weight loss isn't happening as expected, they need to be willing to take a closer look at their diet and perhaps track their food for a couple of days.

Can I advance my diet faster than my surgeon recommends if I feel up to it?

While it can be confusing and disheartening to learn that other surgeons advance the diets of their patients faster than yours does, it is always safest to follow your surgeon's diet. Remember, every surgeon has different surgical techniques and different experiences with patients on which he or she is basing the post-op diet. You chose your surgeon, presumably, because you trusted him or her to offer you the best care. So trust your surgeon and follow his or her advice. Only advance your diet when your surgeon says it's OK and not a moment sooner.

The hardest part for me was the second week of the full liquid diet. At this point, I had been on liquids for about four weeks—two weeks pre-op and two weeks post-op. I really wanted to just eat something different. I was so sick of the shakes that I thought I'd lose my mind. I wasn't hungry; I was just sick of shakes, so I tried to get creative. While on full liquids I was allowed strained soups, so I'd puree some cream of mushroom soup in the blender, strain it through a mesh sieve, and stir in some chicken soup flavored protein powder for some extra protein. Then, at the next meal, I'd try it with a different type of soup or add some different seasonings. Looking back, the liquid phase of my diet passed very quickly but at the time it seemed to last forever.

Just try to be as creative you can within the limits of the diet and know that you'll be advancing your diet soon. Advancing your diet too early can be dangerous and can cause a serious setback in your healing.

When should I plan to return to work?

Speak to your surgeon, and of course be mindful of what your work will allow. Ideally, take off at least one week from a desk job and more if you job requires more physically. You may want to consider taking a week off and then only going back half-days for a few days until you feel ready for a full day.

While employers always understandably want to know exactly how long you will be gone, in truth it is hard to know how long you will take to heal. There are many variables out of your control, such as possible complications, that would necessitate an extension of your absence. Be sure you fully understand your rights as an employee and how much time you will be allowed (paid or unpaid) if needed.

When will I be able to exercise?

You cannot exercise until your surgeon gives you clearance to do so. My surgeon gave me full clearance to exercise at 6 weeks after surgery, although I was encouraged to walk a lot before then.

When can I start to lift heavy things again?

My surgeon told me not to lift more than 10 pounds for 3 weeks and 20 pounds for 6 weeks. This is harder than you may think, especially if you have young kids who need to be lifted into car seats, cribs, high chairs, and sometimes just picked up and hugged! The lifting restriction gets especially hard after about 2 weeks when you feel pretty good but are still not allowed to lift. Try to follow your surgeon's instructions on lifting restrictions. The earlier out your try to lift something the more likely you are to injure yourself.

Will I regret the surgery?

"Buyer's remorse" is a phrase commonly used to describe how patients sometimes feel right after surgery. In this case, they aren't regretting purchasing something frivolous, but they are regretting forcing themselves into a new lifestyle. Buyer's remorse often happens in those first few weeks after surgery when you are still sore, and you are sick of drinking protein shakes. Talk it out with a supportive friend or spouse, or bring it up at your support group. Know that the feeling will pass as your start to lose weight and begin to enjoy the life you've always wanted for yourself. Envision yourself at goal and imagine getting to do all the things you've wanted to do but couldn't because of your weight. Know that this feeling is normal and it will get better. This is a major life adjustment, and it takes time.

Most surgeons have a psychologist on their team or can refer you to one who is experienced in working with weight loss surgery patients. If you feel yourself going beyond the typical "buyer's remorse" and into a situation where you feel depressed or anxious, it's a good idea to check in with a counselor who can help you work through this challenging time. This is especially important if you believe you have issues with food addiction.

Remember—weight loss surgery is surgery on your stomach and not your head. The sleeve, while it significantly reduces hunger and helps you feel full quickly, does NOT take away your urge to eat for non-hunger reasons. If you tend to turn to food when you are stressed, you may feel upset that you are no longer able to do so, and that can certainly make your buyer's remorse grow into something bigger. A good counselor can be a central player in your journey to a healthy new you!

What are the symptoms of a leak?

A leak can occur anytime after surgery. Usually leaks happen within the first two or three weeks, but they can happen anytime before your staple line is fully healed. The hospital should discharge you with instructions on when to call the hospital, including informing you about the signs of a possible leak.

Here are a few possible symptoms of a leak. Keep in mind, you won't likely have every symptom on the list, and you might have some symptoms that aren't on the list at all. Always contact your surgeon's office or the hospital if you are concerned about anything you experience.

- Fever (over 100 degrees)
- Extreme abdominal pain
- Racing heart
- Pain elsewhere, such as the shoulders

Again, if you are ever in doubt about a symptom, always call your surgeon's office right away.

When should I call my surgeon or go to the hospital?

The hospital should discharge you with this information. Follow their instructions for when to call or go back to the hospital. As a general rule, if you are in doubt about *anything*, you should call your surgeon's office. Believe me, your health care providers would rather have a bunch of false alarms than miss one complication that quickly spirals into something worse!

Some sure signs that you need to contact the surgeon include a fever, signs of infection at your incision sites, nausea or vomiting that cannot be controlled, and dehydration. Sometimes, weight loss surgery patients struggle to take in adequate fluids and must return to the hospital for IV fluids. Dehydration can get serious, fast, so it is important to always make drinking liquids a priority.

When will I start to feel "normal" again?

I started to feel pretty normal about two weeks after surgery, although some feel normal sooner and some later. By "normal" I mean that it is easy to forget that I recently had surgery. Be careful, though. When you start to feel well, you might want to instantly resume your normal pre-op activities, but you can't! You have to be mindful of not only your new dietary restrictions, but your lifting and activity restrictions as well.

CHAPTER 10
WHAT IS LIFE LIKE WITH THE SLEEVE?

Once you are fully healed from the surgery, this is when the real work begins. You are now faced with an altered body and a team of professionals, friends, and family all expecting you to lose a lot of weight. It can be overwhelming, but mostly it's an exhilarating time. Some people call this the "honeymoon phase." The first six months after your sleeve surgery is a time when you will see your fastest weight loss.

How much and how quickly you will lose will depend on how much weight you have to lose to begin with, how much you exercise, how strict you are with your diet, your individual metabolism, and other health conditions. I always advise people to use this "honeymoon period" wisely. Follow all the rules. Establish a new lifestyle and new habits. Once the honeymoon is over, your weight loss will come slower, so maximize your weight loss while you can!

How is my goal weight determined?

Patients and surgeons often set different weight goals. Sometimes, the surgeon wants the patient at a lower weight goal than the patient wants, but more often the surgeon sets a higher weight goal than the patient hopes to achieve. It's OK to have your own goal number in mind, but it is important to have discussion with your surgeon about where he or she expects to you to be in 3 months, 6 months, one year, and beyond surgery.

When a surgeon sets a weight goal, it can depend on a number of factors: your starting weight, your BMI, your body composition (such as percent body fat), your weight history, and your age. If you have been super morbidly obese (a BMI over 50) almost your entire adult life, your surgeon may want you to achieve a BMI of 29. A BMI of 29 is still technically overweight, but it is out of the obese category of a 30 BMI or higher, which is where you statistically have a much higher risk of weight related health problems. A BMI of 29 might be a realistic goal for such a patient, and the patient would expect to see major health improvements if he or she reaches this goal as well as an improved quality of life.

A patient with a BMI of 40 who was only morbidly obese for 5 years might have a lower BMI set as a goal. Perhaps the surgeon would expect that this patient could return to a BMI that he or she used to maintain successfully before gaining weight—perhaps a BMI of 23, for example.

Many surgeons use a formula to set your weight goal. This formula typically accounts for the average percent of excess weight loss and might be based on data from the surgeon's own practice, or national data. For instance, suppose a surgeon finds that most of his or her sleeve patients lose 80% of their excess body weight. If you weigh 300 pounds and your ideal weight is 150 pounds, that means you have 150 pounds of excess weight. The surgeon may set a goal for this patient to lose 120 pounds, or 80% of his or her excess weight. This patient's goal weight would be 180 pounds.

Whatever your ultimate goal is, I recommend that you set mini-goals. It will help to keep you motivated and give you many opportunities to celebrate your success along your journey.

How many calories do you eat, on average?

My nutritionist and surgeon's office gave me a suggested range of 600-800 calories per day. On average, during my losing phase, I ate approximately 650 calories per day. I found that eating near the lower end of the range maximized my weight loss. On days where I had extremely strenuous exercise, I would eat more towards the 800-calorie end. Usually, though, 650 was the "magic number" for me to feel good and lose weight quickly.

How much fat/carb/protein do you eat every day?

It isn't just about counting calories; they have to be the *right kind* of calories. The guidelines that my nutritionist provided for me recommended that I eat at least 65 grams of protein and less than 60 grams of carbohydrates per day. On average, I ate about 70 grams of protein and about 40 grams of carbohydrates. I didn't pay very close attention to fat as my diet was relatively low fat. In fact, you *do* need fat in your diet and you might find your hair and skin getting dry if you don't eat enough. My average daily fat intake was about 20 grams, although it varied greatly.

Are there any foods that you can't eat?

This is one of the best features of the sleeve surgery as opposed to the other most popular weight loss surgeries. I don't have to worry about foods making me sick or getting "stuck." In the first 6 weeks, I had to follow my surgeon's diet plan that eased me from a liquid diet to soft foods to regular foods. I also had to wait 3 months before I could eat raw fibrous fruits and vegetables. Other than these restrictions related to healing, there were no official food restrictions. If I wanted a small bite of cake at my daughter's birthday party, I could have it. I didn't have to worry about getting sick with dumping syndrome.

Having said that, though, while I was losing weight I chose NOT to eat a bite of cake at my daughter's birthday party. It just didn't seem worth it to eat all those calories and not have any protein to show for it!

It can be a big adjustment in social situations to not be eating, or to be eating very little, but you'll find that people appreciate someone playing hostess. You can keep busy re-filling peoples glasses of water, clearing dishes, and enjoying conversation. People will adjust to the new you, and you'll adjust to socializing without eating what everyone else is eating too. Now, if you do decide to eat that bite of cake, that's OK. Just be sure to account for it. As long as you are hitting your calorie goals, eating enough protein, and drinking enough water, there is room for little indulgences!

Does food get stuck?

Gastric bypass patients sometimes have problems with food getting stuck between their stomach and their intestines. Adjustable band patients sometimes get food stuck in the area where the band squeezes the stomach into two parts—a small pouch and the rest of the stomach. Sleeve patients (and duodenal switch patients as well) do not have this issue because they have their natural pyloric valve intact.

The pyloric valve, or sphincter, is a ring of muscle that passes food from your stomach to your small intestines. Just as food doesn't get stuck in this valve before surgery, it won't get stuck after surgery either. Still, it is important that you chew your food well. Your smaller stomach can use the extra help in breaking down food into smaller particles for digestion, plus chewing thoroughly will also help you to eat slower which, will help you avoid over-eating.

How much food can you eat in one sitting?

It depends on the size of your sleeve. The size of your sleeve depends on the size of the bougie your surgeon used, how tightly he or she made your sleeve, and the length of your natural stomach. Remember, the sleeve surgery just removes the greater curvature of the stomach. The distance between your esophagus and your pyloric valve can vary depending on your height, build, and genetics, so no two sleeves are exactly alike.

Many patients find they can only eat about 1 ounce of soft food in the early stages. Later, they can eat 2 ounces. By the time they are in maintenance, they can eat 3 or even 4 ounces in a sitting. Again, this is highly individual.

You might find that some foods are "slider foods" in that you seem to be able to eat more of them than other foods. Generally, these are foods to avoid. The purpose of the sleeve is to allow you to feel full on very little food. Seeking out foods that you know are "sliders" defeats the purpose. While I didn't have any slider foods, per se, I did know that I could drink a lot of liquids without getting full. I could easily (probably) drink a big chocolate malt, and it would go through my stomach fast enough that I could eat much more than I should, so, I never even tried.

Are you allowed to eat and drink at the same time?

No, we are advised not to eat and drink at the same time. It won't make most people sick, but it will quickly push food through your stomach, which will allow you to eat more than you should. Some people do report that they get a stomach ache if they drink and eat at the same time, but everyone is different. Sometimes dumping a bunch of water on top of an already over-packed sleeve can lead to an almost instant regurgitation of the water.

Just like the advice to avoid any "slider foods" you may discover, the goal is to maximize the restriction of the sleeve to let it do its job in helping you lose weight. If a patient wanted to, he or she could indeed not lose weight with the sleeve by eating all day, ingesting a lot of liquid calories, or trying to push more food through by drinking while eating, but we got the sleeve to help us lose weight, not to find ways around it! If you find that you are trying to eat more than you should, it's a good idea to call a counselor to work through any underlying issues. The sleeve is a marvelous and powerful tool for weight loss, but you have to use it properly to have success!

Does hunger come back?

For some patients, it does come back; however, for many (myself included, so far) it does not. Even for patients who report that their hunger returns, most say it isn't as powerful as it was before the sleeve surgery. They are better able to manage it; moreover, with a smaller stomach it is easy to satisfy their hunger. Some patients who experience hunger find that taking an acid reducer can minimize what seem to be hunger-pangs but are really just an over-production of acid. If you have problems with hunger, ask your surgeon if he or she thinks an acid reducer might help.

It is also important to note that there is a difference between physical hunger and "head hunger." Most of us are familiar with physical hunger, and certainly anyone reading this book has likely dieted in the past and can tell you what physical hunger feels like after eating celery all day! Head hunger, however, is very different. It can feel as real as and even more intense than physical hunger, but its origins are psychological rather than physical. If you are an emotional eater or if you believe you have a food addiction, it is important to understand that the sleeve surgery will not automatically fix these issues. When you decide to move ahead with weight loss surgery, you have to fully commit yourself to the process of changing your lifestyle and your outlook on food. The issues of head hunger are best addressed with a professional counselor, especially one with experience working with weight loss surgery patients or eating disorders.

I've said it before, and I'll say it again. The sleeve is surgery on your stomach and not your head! Don't neglect to deal with any head issues that you might have as they relate to food and your health!

Do sleeve patients frequently develop GERD?

Studies on GERD and the sleeve appear to be inconsistent (Chiu, Birch, Shi, Sharma, Karmali. 2011.

Effect of sleeve gastrectomy on gastroesophageal reflux disease: A systematic review. Surgery for Obesity and Related Diseases **7**, 500-5); however, my surgeon told me that he does see many cases of acid reflux in his sleeve patients. It has been speculated that the smaller and tighter the sleeve, the greater the likelihood that GERD will occur; however, there are no solid scientific studies to support this hypothesis.

In any case, I did develop GERD. I had only had heartburn one time in my life prior to sleeve surgery, and that was when I was pregnant. I experienced a burning sensation in my throat and base of my neck. I asked my surgeon about it he prescribed a proton-pump inhibitor (PPI). One small pill a day is all I need, and I haven't had any acid problems since.

Some patients report that they feel hungrier when they have too much acid in their stomach, and they say that a PPI significantly reduces the feelings of hunger.

Do you tell people that you had the sleeve?

I shared my plans for sleeve surgery with my family and my closest friends. All were extremely supportive and enthusiastic, and I know I am very fortunate to have received such great responses. With neighbors, business associates, and other acquaintances I tend to be more guarded. If someone asks me how I've lost weight, I can honestly tell them that I'm eating less and exercising more. If the someone asks me directly, or if someone has a weight problem and wants to know the details of how I did it – I tell them!

Some people in my support group tell anyone and everyone, whether they want to hear about it or not, that they've had weight loss surgery. Others have told no one except for their spouse or significant other. It's a personal matter, so there is no right or wrong.

The more people you tell, the more you open yourself up to discouraging opinions. Believe me, *everyone* has an opinion on weight loss surgery! Some people enjoy debating others on it, some don't. I don't feel at all ashamed of my decision. I'm proud that I took charge of my obesity and made my life better using the best tools that modern medicine could offer, but, does my postman need to know about it? Probably not, but if he ever asks, I'll gladly tell him.

There is one thing to consider when deciding how open to be about your weight loss surgery. While this lifestyle change is forever, the "losing phase" of your new life is brief. It's while you are losing weight that people will be asking a lot of questions. Once you are at goal weight, you'll just be seen as an average (or even small) person who eats lightly and exercises. The longer you are in maintenance, the more you'll realize that no one really cares or notices what you are or are not eating. Very few people will ever ask you "Have you ever been morbidly obese?" The sleeve will always be part of your life, but it won't always feel like it is center stage as it does the first 6 months or year after your surgery. So if you are at all uncertain about whether or not you want to share with someone that you voluntarily removed 85% of your stomach, always remember that you cannot "untell" them.

How do you stay motivated?

When you are in the losing phase, it is easy to stay motivated with regular weigh-ins. Once a week is a good standard for how often you should weigh yourself. If you weigh yourself daily (something we've all done from time to time) you might make yourself crazy with inevitable fluctuations in water weight that might make the scale hop up a pound from time to time. Weighing in once a week and seeing the numbers drop will give you the drive to keep going.

Also, don't forget to take some measurements before your surgery. When you go through an inevitable weight loss stall, it's a good time to take out the tape measure and see how much smaller you are getting—even if the number on the scale is being temporarily stubborn. Measure your chest, waist, hips, thighs, calves, neck, and upper arms. You might need a trusted partner to help make some of the measurements, but they will be well worth it to have as a motivator for later!

As you lose weight, take pictures to document your loss. Nothing will motivate you more than seeing your picture at your highest weight and comparing it to a picture from 1 month, 2 months, 3 months, and further out from your surgery. Some patients in my support group even like to carry a "before" picture of themselves in their wallets. Anytime they need some extra motivation, they take a look at it.

What happens if you "cheat" on your diet with the sleeve?

There can be serious consequences if you advance your diet too quickly or eat too much early after surgery. You could even end up in the hospital, or worse. Take your surgeon's dietary guidelines seriously and protect that tender staple line of your new stomach. No food is worth risking your healing. Once you are healed, the main consequences of eating the wrong foods are really just slowing or halting your weight loss. Unlike gastric bypass patients, sleeve patients do not experience dumping syndrome if they eat something that is too fatty or too sugary. If you eat too much of any food, you might throw up. Many sleeve patients accidentally overeat as they are learning how much their stomach can hold. This is why it's always a good idea to measure your food. If you know you cannot eat more than 2 ounces of cheese for a snack, then measure out 2 ounces of cheese.

Can the sleeve get stretched out?

Sleeve capacity does *seem* to increase the further out from surgery you get, but only to a point. Initially, after surgery, you will have a lot of swelling in your stomach, which will limit your capacity greatly. As the swelling dissipates, you will have an increased capacity, but this is *not* due to stretching.

Ideally, most sleeves are made from the least stretchy part of the original stomach. The fundus, the stretchy part of the stomach that expands when we eat a big meal and can eventually get stretched out, is removed. Unlike the pouch of the gastric bypass patient, the sleeve should not have any portion of the fundus remaining. There is anecdotal evidence that the smaller the sleeve is initially, the less chance it will have of stretching later; however, there is no scientific evidence to date verifying if this is true. If you always eat just *under* your sleeves maximum capacity, you never have to worry about vomiting from overeating, and you will also won't need to worry about stretching your sleeve.

How do I know the sleeve would work for me?

Many weight loss surgery patients have the fear that the surgery will not work for them. In fact, patients *do* fail to lose enough weight with the sleeve and fail to keep it off just like patients fail with every type of weight loss surgery. The majority of sleeve patients succeed, however, and if you care enough about your success that you are reading this book, I think they odds are that you will be one of those success stories too! The sleeve is a tool, a powerful tool, but not a magic wand. You have to follow the rules and work hard to ensure your success. Not only during the weight loss phase of your journey, but also during maintenance. If you follow the rules, you will lose the weight and keep it off.

What if I don't lose all my weight during the "honeymoon period"?

While my surgeon and my support group put great emphasis on taking advantage of the "honeymoon period" you should know that there is nothing magical about it. Your body doesn't really know the difference between being 5 months and 28 days out from surgery versus 6 months and 2 days. Patients can, and often do, continue to lose weight after the 6-month mark. The reason the honeymoon period is so important is because the weight loss is faster and easier at first. If you just glide through this period effortlessly, without establishing new healthy habits (such as exercise and food tracking), then you are less likely to continue losing or to keep the weight off successfully. It's not impossible, but it is harder to establish new habits later rather than doing it right away.

Take these 6 months as a time to readjust your entire lifestyle. Learn some new exercise routines and make them part of your daily life. Learn more about nutrition. Work with a counselor on any emotional eating issues or food addictions that might pose a barrier to your long terms success. That way, when your weight loss slows down (which it inevitably will; you can't keep losing weight forever!) you will be living a healthy lifestyle that will enable you to lose any remaining weight and keep it off. If you don't establish these healthy habits, you may find yourself unable to take off the last few pounds or struggling to maintain your weight loss.

Having said all of that, don't get too hung up on the concept of a honeymoon phase. If you have a bad day, or even a bad week, you can always get back on track no matter where you are in your weight loss journey. If you have more than 200 pounds to lose, you might even lose more weight after the honeymoon phase than you did during the honeymoon phase! The main point is, establish a new lifestyle right away. Don't just coast on the "easy weight loss" you might experience in the beginning. You are in this *for life*!

How do you deal with weight loss stalls?

Weight loss stalls are almost inevitable. When I was about 6 weeks out from surgery, I hit a stall that lasted almost 3 weeks. I was doing everything right. I was eating 650 calories a day, getting in my protein and water, and exercising, but still the scale wouldn't budge. I visited the nutritionist and asked her what I was doing wrong. She just smiled and said, "Nothing, sometime it seems as if our bodies just need a break." While her response wasn't entirely satisfying, I knew I was doing everything I could to stay on the program. She told me that it would break, and I'd start losing again. She was right.

By the time I had finally started losing weight again, I had gained a new appreciation for the sleeve. You see, without the sleeve, if I were just dieting on my own and hit a major stall like this, I would have just thrown up my hands and said "See? Diets don't work for me!" Then, I would have gone back to my old eating habits and likely gained back all the weight I had lost. This time was different. This time I had the sleeve in my corner and it kept me strong. It helped me to not cheat; it helped me to stay on track. The stall ended with me *losing* weight, not with me *gaining* weight because I had given up. I was very grateful for the sleeve.

When you hit a stall in your weight loss journey, there are many tricks that people try to employ to break them. You might change your exercise routine. You might try lowering, or even increasing, your calorie intake. You may want to increase your water and protein intake. Whatever you do, I would advise you to just make sure it is within the parameters of the diet plan laid out for you by your surgeon and nutritionist. Don't turn your body into a science experiment. If you stick with the program, you can at least know you are doing everything right to stay on track. If you start to stray too far from the plan, even if it's in an earnest effort to break a stall, it may be hard to come back. Have patience, tweak your exercise routines, take some measurements to remind yourself that you are losing inches, and stay the course. If you still have weight to lose, you will eventually lose it.

How many vitamins do you have to take every day?

Even though sleeve patients aren't fighting against the malabsorption of vitamins that gastric bypass patients deal with, we still need to take vitamins in order to ensure we are getting what we need every day. Our highly restricted food intake makes it almost impossible to get all of our recommended daily allowances through food alone.

Many sleeve patients, me included, use a protein shake every day to help ensure they get enough protein. I also take a multi-vitamin, B-12, iron, D-3, and calcium. Every patient has different needs, though, and my vitamin regimen isn't the same as what your vitamin regimen may need to be. Your surgeon will advise you on what vitamins you need to take and when to start taking them. Many vitamins can wait until you are fully healed from your surgery. You should also have regular blood tests to catch any deficiencies that might need to be corrected.

How much exercise do you have to do to be successful?

You can certainly lose weight without exercising. The majority of weight that you lose is from cutting calories in your diet rather than calories burned during exercise, but, exercise has a lot of benefits. It keeps you healthy and strong. It will help you sleep better at night. As you build muscle, it will also improve your resting metabolic rate, which will allow you to eat a few more calories every day while in maintenance.

Once you are cleared for exercise, it is best to start slow. If your program offers a personal trainer, take advantage of this opportunity to learn how to exercise properly and with maximum benefit. Three times a week for at least 30 minutes is a good place to start. If you can work your way up to 5 times a week, that's even better.

As you lose weight, you'll find that you can do more active things easily. You'll find yourself naturally being more active throughout the day. You won't think anything of taking the stairs rather than an elevator. You might walk down the street to the grocery store rather than driving like you did in the past. You'll be burning more calories just by being a more active person, beyond the exercise program you develop.

Whatever you do, try to find at least 2 or 3 different workouts that you truly enjoy. Variety will help keep you from getting bored and also help you to exercise different muscle groups. If you think the exercise is fun, you'll be much more likely to stick with it. Getting an exercise buddy can also be a great motivator and help get you off the couch on days that you'd otherwise let your workout slide.

How much weight should I expect to lose with the sleeve?

This is the big question! Recent studies have shown that weight loss with the sleeve is very similar to weight loss with the gastric bypass. In fact, the Updated Position Statement on the Sleeve Gastrectomy as a Bariatric Procedure by the American Society for Metabolic and Bariatric Surgery (ASMBS) published in October 2011 states that the new literature generally shows "equivalence or superiority" of the sleeve to gastric bypass or adjustable gastric banding in the short and medium term. No wonder so many think the sleeve is going to become the new "gold standard" of weight loss surgery some day! Everyone is anxious for the day when more long-term data can be provided and hopeful that this trend will continue.

The same statement from the ASMBS refers to data from the 3rd International Summit for Sleeve Gastrectomy, which included data provided by 88 surgeons performing over 19,000 sleeve gastrectomies. The mean percentage of excess weight loss reported was 62.7% at 1 year, 64.7% at 2 years, 64% at 3 years, 57.3% at 4 years, and 60.0% at 5 years.

What does this data mean to you? If you are 150 pounds overweight (meaning 150 pounds above your healthy weight as determined by BMI) and you lose an "average" amount of weight, you can expect to lose 62% of 150 lbs in the first year, which is 92 pounds. Keep in mind, though, that these are averages. Some patients lose more and some patients lose less. What is exciting is that these initial reports seem to indicate that sleeve patients *keep the weight off.*

Now that your head is likely spinning with statistics, I will tell you that my surgeon said 10 pounds a month is a good goal for most sleeve patients. You'll probably lose a bit more than that early on, and a less as you get closer to your goal.

How long will it take me to lose all my excess weight with the sleeve?

It depends on how much you have to lose, as well as many other variables. If you have 100 pounds to lose, and you lose an average of 10 pounds a month, you will lose all your excess weight in 10 months. If you have 200 lbs or more to lose, it could take you 2 years before you reach your goal. Everyone is different.

What if I stop losing weight before I reach my goal?

As you get closer to your goal, you will likely find that your weight loss slows down. It might even stop, or at least hit a really long plateau, short of reaching your goal. If this happens, there are several things to consider.

First, is it possible that your body has reached its healthy weight? Sometimes it is difficult to set realistic goals, especially if you have been obese for most of your adult life. Some people naturally have higher body weights than others. It can depend on your bone structure and muscle mass. Perhaps the last time you were at a healthy weight, you were 16 years old. It isn't realistic to expect that a 50-year-old body is going to settle on the same healthy weight as a 16-year-old body. Talk to your surgeon, or your physician, if you think you may need to reassess your goal weight. You might be surprised that your body is healthy and happy at a healthy weight at 150 pounds instead of the 130 pounds that you hoped to weigh.

Second, if you've lost a great deal of weight there is a good chance you have some excess skin. Some patients find they are unable to reach their goal weight due to excess skin. You will have to decide if you want to have plastic surgery to remove it or if you will readjust your expectations for your final weight.

Third, if the above two factors do not apply to you, it could be that you need to push a bit harder, or change some things in your diet and exercise program in order to get those last few pounds off. Some patients find success by "returning to basics." They go back to their protein shakes and cut calories to the bottom of the range recommended by their nutritionist. You may also want to try changing your exercise routine. If you usually walk, try swimming. If you usually do kickboxing, try step aerobics. Changing your exercise routine will change the muscles that you use and increase your calorie burn.

No matter how you decide to change things to get those last few pounds off, I definitely recommend that you return to counting and measuring everything. If you've gotten out of the habit of measuring and writing down everything you eat, you might be surprised by just how many calories you are taking in every day. Sometimes the simple act of tracking all your food intake can melt away those last few pounds!

CHAPTER 11
WHAT SHOULD I EXPECT IN MAINTENANCE?

Obese people cannot eat the same way that naturally thin people do. I know, life isn't fair—right? This is extremely important to know and understand, however. Even though you are now the same weight as your naturally thin friends, it doesn't mean that you can eat like them and stay thin! Obesity changes our bodies in significant ways. Your metabolism will never be the same as a naturally thin person. You will need to eat less and exercise more in order to maintain a healthy weight.

What does a maintenance diet look like?

Once you have reached your goal weight, you can slowly begin to add more calories to your diet. The slower you increase your calories the better as it will help you to determine the right calorie level to maintain your weight.

Fortunately, your sleeve is a tool for life! It will help you to continue to eat smaller portions, even after you've reached your goal weight. You should continue to follow all the rules of healthy eating— eat protein first, drink lots of water, take your vitamins, avoid overly processed foods, etc. If you were eating 600-800 calories a day while you were losing weight, you might find you are eating 1000-1200 calories a day in maintenance. The exact calories will depend on your activity level and individual metabolism. Some tall athletic men can consume up to 2000 or more calories a day and maintain their goal weight. It is highly individual. Remember that you can continue to use your surgeon and nutritionist as a resource, even after you've reached your goal. They can help guide you in developing a maintenance plan.

Perhaps the most important thing you can do in maintenance is continue to weigh yourself regularly. Every week or every other week should be adequate. Decide on a small range that is acceptable for your weight. For example, if you reached your goal weight of 160, give yourself a 6-pound cushion for weight fluctuations. As long as you weight stays between 157 and163 pounds, you are in good shape. If your weight creeps down too low or too high, it's time to immediately start tracking your food intake again and see where you need to make changes. By staying on top of your weight, you can ensure that you will never return to the morbidly obese person you were before sleeve surgery.

Do you still have as much restriction in maintenance as you did while losing weight?

The sleeve is not expected to stretch very much over time because it is made from the least stretchy part of the stomach. You *will* continue to have restriction; however, just like when you had a pre-sleeved stomach, you can always push yourself beyond what is comfortable. It is entirely possible to graze all day on unhealthy foods and gain weight with the sleeve. So stick to an eating schedule, eating three meals a day and two small snacks and nothing more. Most sleeve patients find they have just as much restriction at 1, 2, and 3 years out from surgery as they did at 6 months out from surgery.

Do you still have to keep track of your food intake during maintenance?

Some patients do, but many do not. It depends on what makes you comfortable. By the time you reach maintenance, you should have established healthy eating habits and an active lifestyle that will help you maintain your weight. Many patients enjoy the fact that they don't need to track their food anymore to know that they are eating properly. No matter what you choose, it is critical that you always monitor your weight. If your weight goes beyond a certain point (usually a few pounds above your goal weight) then you need to start tracking food again and see if you are taking in more calories than you realize. While maintenance is much more relaxed and you can treat yourself occasionally, you will always have to vigilant about your weight for the rest of your life to avoid regaining your lost weight.

Do you ever feel hungry?

Some sleeve patients report that hunger returns, but many say it does not. You might have "head hunger," which is related to psychological reasons that you wish to eat. You might have excess stomach acid, which mimics the feeling of hunger, but with your smaller stomach and the dramatic decrease in the hormone ghrelin, hunger as you knew it as a pre-op will most likely be a thing of the past.

Are you "allowed" to eat treats—such as a piece of birthday cake?

One of the reasons I chose the sleeve was that I didn't want any foods to be off limits for the rest of my life. With the sleeve, you don't have to worry about getting sick with "dumping syndrome" if you eat something high in carbs or simple sugars. While it's best to avoid any sweets while in the losing phase of your weight loss journey, there is room for the occasional treat while in maintenance. The treats should be few and far between and reserved for special occasions. If you are generally eating healthy, low calorie foods and exercising, then you should be able to fit occasional treats into your maintenance plan!

There are some weight loss surgery patients who struggle with food addiction. For these patients, having "just one bite" of cake or another sweet could trigger them to binge on much more. Only you know what you can handle. For patients working through food addiction issues, sometimes it's better to just not "go there."

Do you continue to go to support group after you are done losing weight?

Yes, support group is a great way to keep your head in the game. It's an opportunity to learn new things, make friends, and offer support to others who are just beginning the journey. If you have enjoyed going to support group during your weight loss, I'd recommend that you continue to go during maintenance. Most support groups have an open door policy. Even if you stopped going for a while, you can always re-join. We often have people coming to our group who had weight loss surgery several years in the past. Some come back to share their success, and some come back seeking support because they have gained some weight. Everyone is welcome!

Do many sleeve patients regain the weight they lost?

While there aren't any long-term studies (10 or more years) at this time, initial short and medium term data look excellent. The statement from the ASMBS refers to data from the 3rd International Summit for Sleeve Gastrectomy, which included data provided by 88 surgeons performing over 19,000 sleeve gastrectomies. The mean percentage of excess weight loss reported was 62.7% at 1 year, 64.7% at 2 years, 64% at 3 years, 57.3% at 4 years, and 60.0% at 5 years. As you can see, 62.7% lost at 1 year and 60.0% at 5 years; these percentages are very similar. This does show that sleeve patients appear to be keeping off most the weight they lose even five years after surgery.

As with any weight loss surgery, however, some patients can and do regain weight. It isn't unusual to regain a few pounds from your lowest weight as your body settles at a healthy weight. In fact, some surgeons recommend that their patients lose a few extra pounds beyond their goal weight to account for this almost inevitable rebound.

Once you are settled at a healthy weight, you will always need to be vigilant and weigh yourself regularly. Be prepared to take action the moment it starts to creep up.

Do many patients lose their hair after losing weight?

Hair loss is pretty common. Many patients lose hair in the first year after surgery, although some may lose it later. I personally started to lose a lot of hair about 3 months after surgery. I never had a bald spot, but I could pull out small fistfuls just by running my fingers through my hair.

At the recommendation of a nurse in my bariatric program, I began to take biotin. Biotin is an over-the-counter supplement that is supposed to help hair, nail, and skin health. I honestly couldn't tell much of a difference after taking biotin, but I continued to take the pill every day while I was in the losing phase. Some patients say it helps while others can't tell much difference.

In any case, you should know that hair loss is almost always temporary. Speak to your surgeon if you have concerns about the amount of hair you are losing, as he or she might have some suggestions specific to your situation. In the meantime, make sure you're eating a healthy diet with lots of protein and water and take your vitamins.

Do patients get left with a lot of extra skin? Does the skin ever shrink?

The more weight you have to lose, the more likely you are to be stuck with extra skin once your reach your goal weight. The older you are, the more likely skin is to be an issue. The longer you were obese, the more likely skin is to be an issue. Skin can stretch, and it can "shrink" or rebound to some degree, but if you go from weighing 350 pounds to 150 pounds, well... your skin cannot shrink *that* much.

Some weight loss surgery patients are unhappy with their end results because they didn't realize they would be left with excess skin. Excess skin is usually a cosmetic issue; however, it can also be a medical issue. Rashes and skin deterioration can cause a great deal of discomfort. Sometimes, skin can even become infected.

There are many great products out there to help you cover-up, smooth out, and "hold in" extra skin. Spanx® is a popular line of products that can help smooth your silhouette. If your extra skin makes you self-conscious, you'll become skilled at the art of creative dressing to cover a sagging stomach and batwing arms. In spite of the problems, most sleeve patients will tell you that they'd rather have the extra skin than the extra fat!

When is plastic surgery an option to remove extra skin?

Plastic surgery can remove extra skin, tighten muscles, and lift sagging body parts. Most weight loss surgery patients who reach goal weight would likely qualify from some type of plastic surgery, if they were willing to pay for it out-of-pocket. Plastic surgery is rarely covered by insurance.

Patients who have a lot of rashes, infections, or other medical issues caused by their excess skin can sometimes get insurance approval for certain procedures. The most commonly approved plastic surgery is a panniculectomy—removal of a "panni." A panni is the hanging belly, which often gets rashes and infections due to moisture and rubbing. Removing the panni can alleviate these problems, but the result isn't always as aesthetically pleasing as a tummy tuck.

If you hope to have insurance help cover your plastic surgery, it is important that you document any and all medical issues related to excess skin as soon as you can. Make appointments with your doctor or surgeon when you have rashes or other problems due to your excess skin so it can be documented. Find a plastic surgeon who is willing to work with insurance companies (because some are and some aren't).

Popular plastic surgery procedures for weight loss surgery patients with excess skin include the following: panniculectomy, arm lift, neck lift, tummy tuck, lower body lift, thigh lift, and breast lift and/or augmentation.

CHAPTER 12
A FINAL WORD: SLEEVE RULES TO LIVE BY

As I say throughout this book, I am not a doctor or a medical professional. I am simply a patient who is fighting obesity with the use of a powerful bariatric procedure called the vertical sleeve. Along the way, I've learned some rules for success. I learned these through my own experience, from other patients, and from bariatric professionals.

(1) Eat *less than* full capacity

(2) Never eat and drink at the same time

(3) Exercise 4-6 times a week

(4) Keep carbs low, but not too low (around 40-50 grams a day)

(5) Eat protein first and eat lots of it (at least 60 grams a day)

(6) Drink a lot of water, always have a water bottle with you

(7) Allow 20-30 minutes for a meal (no more, no less)

Good luck in your journey to better health!

80030143R00078

Made in the USA
San Bernardino, CA
22 June 2018